Understanding Colon Cancer

Understanding Health and Sickness Series
Miriam Bloom, Ph.D.
General Editor

Understanding Colon Cancer

A. Richard Adrouny, M.D., F.A.C.P.

University Press of Mississippi
Jackson

7/12

www.upress.state.ms.us

Copyright © 2002 by University Press of Mississippi
All rights reserved
Manufactured in the United States of America
Illustrations by Alan Estridge

10   09   08   07   06   05   04   03   02   4   3   2   1
∞

Library of Congress Cataloging-in-Publication Data

Adrouny, A. Richard, 1952–
     Understanding colon cancer / A. Richard Adrouny.
        p.; cm. — (Understanding health and sickness series)
     Includes bibliographical references and index.
     ISBN 1-57806-472-4 (cloth : alk. paper)—ISBN 1-57806-473-2
(paper : alk. paper)
     1. Colon (Anatomy)—Cancer—Popular works. [DNLM: 1. Colonic
Neoplasms—etiology. 2. Colonic Neoplasms—prevention & control.
3. Colonic Neoplasms—therapy. WI529 A243u 2002] I. Title. II. Series.
RC280.C6 A35 2002
616.99'4347—dc21   2002000788

British Library Cataloging-in-Publication Data available

Contents

Acknowledgments

I received help from many people during the preparation
of this book. Mr. Mike Liddicoat, M.L.I.S., of the Community
Health Library of Los Gatos generously gave his time to
obtain reprints of articles that I used in my research. My
colleagues Richard S. Coughlin, M.D. (colorectal surgery),
Robert Filpi, M.D. (radiology), S. Robert Freedman, M.D.
(pathology), Wallace Sampson, M.D. (medical oncology),
and Mark M. Segall, M.D. (colorectal surgery), were kind
enough to review portions of the book and provide useful
criticism. Dick Coughlin allowed me to use his compilation of
screening guidelines and recommendations; Bob Filpi also
provided me with illustrative x-rays and useful articles on
the radiology of colon cancer; similarly, Robert B. Abing-
ton, M.D. (nuclear medicine), was kind enough to give me
a folder of reprints on PET scanning and nuclear scintigraphy. Mahendra Ranchod, M.D. (pathology), kindly provided
me with photographs of colon cancer specimens from his
pathology teaching files, and Mark Segall provided me with
endoscopic photographs of colon cancer from his patient files.
Photographs have also been obtained from my own patient
files. Other illustrations are acknowledged in the text.

This book would not have been written had I not been
asked by Miriam Bloom, Ph.D., to do it. I am grateful for her
guiding hand along the way.

I am grateful for the privilege of having been physician
to so many wonderful patients who have given me my truest
education in medicine.

My wife, Karen, and children, Melissa and Greg, have
shown great patience with me, as I have monopolized use
of the family computer and kept articles and books strewn
throughout the study for months while getting this project
completed.

Finally, I would like to dedicate this book to the memory of my father and first teacher of science, George Adour Adrouny, Ph.D., who died during the writing of the manuscript. As professor of biochemistry at Tulane University School of Medicine, he touched the lives of many students. From him I learned not only biochemistry but also the value of perseverance, intellectual curiosity and honesty, and a lasting love and respect for language, especially word origins, clear thinking, and clear writing.

Introduction

Audrey Hepburn. Ronald Reagan. "Tip" O'Neill. Eric Davis. Darryl Strawberry. Charles Schulz. Jay Monahan. Vince Lombardi. All of these famous people, and hundreds of thousands of ordinary people, have had it. "It," of course, is colorectal cancer.

Colorectal cancer is a significant health problem in the United States and the rest of the western world. It is the third most common cause of cancer worldwide. In the United States, it is the second most common cause of cancer in both men and women. However, the public is not as well acquainted with this disease as it should be. While colorectal cancer has been quietly ignored for decades, other cancers, including cancer of the lung, breast, ovary, and prostate, have been grabbing headlines for years. However, the image of colon cancer languishing in medical awareness purgatory is slowly beginning to change.

The public is becoming aware of the value of screening for this disease. While breast cancer can be detected early by mammography and prostate cancer by PSA (prostate specific antigen) blood testing, colon cancer can be detected in its premalignant or asymptomatic stages when prevention or cure is possible. (Note: in this book, the terms *colon, colorectal, large bowel,* and *large intestine* are used interchangeably, although when the discussion concerns distinct regions of the large intestine, the colon is distinguished from the rectum.)

The advent of fiberoptic endoscopy in recent decades has reformed our way of thinking about the disease and has provided unprecedented intelligence about its natural history. Colorectal cancer can be viewed as a disease confined to a geometrically and anatomically distinct plane of tissue that is readily accessible to direct examination. Therefore, prospects for elimination of the disease exist in a not too distant realm. Indeed, the incidence of colorectal cancer has declined in recent years, probably because of screening and early diagnosis of potentially malignant polyps.

This book begins with a review of the demographics of colon and rectal cancer and high-risk conditions for the disease. The polyp-to-carcinoma sequence (key to understanding this disease) is explained, along with the polyposis syndromes. The normal anatomy and physiology of the colon is next reviewed, followed by a discussion of colon carcinogenesis. Important information about the genetics of the disease, much of which was uncovered in seminal research of the 1990s, is given in chapter 3.

The "look" (signs) and "feel" (symptoms) of colon cancer are covered next. The importance of symptoms such as bleeding, abdominal pain, and change of bowel habits is reviewed, followed by a look at the important tests useful for the diagnosis and staging of the disease. The stages of colon cancer are then summarized, including discussion of the prognosis according to each stage and theories of how colon cancer spreads.

Treatment of colon cancer is discussed in two chapters, including surgical approaches to the disease according to where in the large bowel the cancer lies, and then review of adjuvant therapies (treatments given in addition to surgery) and treatment of advanced disease with chemotherapy. Laparoscopic surgery is given considerable attention, although it is not yet clear exactly what role this form of surgery will have in the future.

In the next chapter, I review strategies for early detection and prevention of the disease. Standard approaches such as digital rectal examination, fecal occult blood testing, and endoscopy for early detection are discussed, along with recommendations concerning use of these tests for screening. Various preventive strategies such as diet, vitamins, and drugs are also covered, as are recommendations regarding genetic screening.

I conclude with a look at developing diagnostic tests such as "virtual colonoscopy" and developing therapies such as vaccines and monoclonal antibodies, and provide additional information about genetic markers and screening, as well as potential genetic therapies.

A number of original and review articles on the disease were drawn upon as references. Major text chapters which provided valuable general information include "Adenocarcinoma of the Colon and Rectum" by Glenn Steele, Jr., Joel Tepper, Bina T. Motwani, and Howard W. Bruckner in *Cancer Medicine* (Third Edition), edited by James F. Holland, Emil Frei III, Robert C. Bast, Jr., Donald W. Kufe, Donald L. Morton, and Ralph R. Wiechselbaum, and "Colon Cancer" by Alfred M. Cohen, Bruce D. Minsky, and Richard L. Schilsky in *Cancer: Principles and Practice of Oncology* (Fourth Edition), edited by Vincent T. DeVita, Jr., Samuel Hellman, and Steven Rosenberg. The chapter "Colorectal Cancer" by Glenn Steele, Jr., in *Cancer Surgery* (edited by Robert J. McKenna, Sr., and Gerald P. Murphy) provides superb discussion on general aspects of the disease as well as specific issues, such as laparoscopic procedures and sphincter-saving operations. *Gastrointestinal Oncology,* edited by James D. Ahlgren and John S. Macdonald, provides several very illuminating chapters on the subject, particularly the chapter "Colorectal Cancer: Surgical Approach" by Lee E. Smith.

Excellent reviews of colorectal anatomy, physiology, and pathology are to be found in "The Small and Large Intestine" by Jerry S. Trier, Charles L. Krone, and Marvin H. Sleisenger in *Gastrointestinal Disease* (Third Edition), edited by Marvin H. Sleisenger and John S. Fordtran; *The Large Intestine,* edited by Sidney F. Phillips, John H. Pemberton, and Roy G. Shorter; *Diseases of the Colon, Rectum and Anal Canal,* edited by Joseph B. Kirsner and Roy G. Shorter; and *Morson and Dawson's Gastrointestinal Pathology* (Third Edition) by Basil C. Morson, Ian M. P. Dawson, David W. Day, Jeremy R. Jass, Ashley B. Price, and Geraint T. Williams.

Understanding Colon Cancer

I. Who Gets Colon Cancer and Why

Putting the Problem in Perspective

Although there is data to show that colorectal cancer incidence and mortality have been waning in recent decades, cancers of the colon and rectum still cause approximately 40,000 deaths in America annually. There are about 140,000 new cases diagnosed each year. In comparison, about 182,000 women each year are diagnosed with breast cancer, and about 164,000 men and women each year are diagnosed with lung cancer. A total of 180,000 men are diagnosed with prostate cancer annually. In total, about 1.2 million new cases of all types of cancer are diagnosed annually, so it is evident that colon cancer constitutes a large portion, a little more than 10 percent, of the cancer problem in the United States, and is the fourth most frequent type of cancer. As an overall cause of cancer mortality, colorectal cancers are second only to lung cancer. For women, however, colon cancer ranks third behind lung and breast cancer as a cause of mortality, and, for men, it ranks third behind lung and prostate.

The lifetime risk of colorectal cancer in the general population is 2.5 to 5 percent. This means that twenty-five to fifty out of one thousand people will get colon cancer in their lifetimes. This risk is increased two- or threefold if there is a first-degree relative (parent, sibling, or child) who has had an adenomatous polyp or cancer.

Colon cancer occurs twice as often in developed countries than in developing countries, with the highest rates being found in North America, Europe, Australia, and New Zealand. The incidence of colon cancer in Japan has been rising steadily since the end of World War II. The lowest incidence rates are found in Africa and India.

Both hereditary and environmental factors are important in causing the disease. The majority of colon cancer cases are considered to be sporadic, that is, occurring predominantly under the influence of environmental factors. However, there are distinct genetic syndromes that may predispose a person to colon cancer. A small percentage of colon cancer cases are believed to be due to these hereditary conditions (see below).

Sex and Age

Colon cancer shows perhaps only a small sexual bias, as men are affected slightly more by this disease than women. The male:female ratio varies from 1.0 to 1.4 depending on the tumor registry that is reporting the data. Rectal cancer, however, is much more common in men than women.

The risk of colon cancer increases with age. The majority of cases occur in people over the age of sixty. In people between the ages of forty and fifty years the incidence of colorectal cancer is fifteen new cases per hundred thousand persons, while in persons more than eighty years of age the incidence rises to more than four hundred new cases per hundred thousand.

Colorectal cancer in the young (under age twenty) accounts for less than 1 percent of all cases. In this age group, the incidence rate is far higher in blacks than in whites (the opposite of what occurs in adults). The young group of patients tends to have a remarkably high incidence of a particular type of colorectal cancer known as mucinous (which means that the cancer produces mucin, the major component of mucus, in large quantities). Diet does not seem to be a factor, since exposure to potential carcinogens is short (compared to the length of time which adults over the age of fifty have had). Polyposis (growths in the bowel which may later become cancer) are not a factor either. The youngest case of colon cancer ever reported was in a nine-month-old baby.

Although breast cancer seems to attract more attention than colon cancer as a women's health care issue, it is of interest to note that for a woman of age sixty-five, the risk of colorectal cancer nearly equals the risk of breast cancer. Concern has been raised that the high morbidity and mortality of colorectal cancer in women is grossly underappreciated by the general public. This is reflected by surveys of women that have shown that compliance by women with colorectal screening tests was much lower than for breast cancer. For example, less than 24 percent of women over the age of fifty had had sigmoidoscopy (examination of the lower portion of the colon with a sigmoidoscope instrument), while nearly 50 percent had had mammography and more than 50 percent had been screened for cervical cancer. There is more focused attention on breast, ovarian, and cervical cancer than on colorectal cancer in women, leading some to suggest that the public perception is that colorectal cancer is "a man's disease," when in fact it is not.

Women who take hormone replacement therapy (estrogen or estrogen and progesterone) in their postmenopausal years derive benefit from it as a protection against colorectal cancer. One study suggested that the risk of colorectal cancer was cut in half after five to ten years of hormone therapy. It has been suggested that women who take hormone replacement therapy (HRT) may have healthier behaviors in general and may be more likely to have regular medical examinations, including screening tests for early colon cancer detection. But HRT may be beneficial through biochemical and cellular mechanisms. HRT may reduce production of bile acids (by-products of fat digestion), which are thought to have colon-cancer-promoting effects, and may directly prevent or reduce colon cancer cell growth by a variety of other means.

Diet, Environment, and Heredity

Evidence suggests that the main environmental factor is diet. Other environmental exposures, such as smoking, are likely to be involved in causing colon cancer but are not as well documented or understood. Diets having a higher composition of cereal fiber (fiber is composed of plant cellulose and hemicellulose, which provide structural integrity to the cell walls of plants), fruits, and vegetables are thought to reduce the risk of colon cancer, while diets high in fat intake and low in fiber are thought to increase the risk. Thus in geographic areas such as Asia and Africa where dietary customs place emphasis on low-fat, high-fiber foods, fruits, and vegetables, people have lower incidence of colon cancer than in the United States and Europe. The exact reason (or reasons) for the protective effect of cereal fiber is not known. Among the most credible theories may be the dilutional effect that fiber bulk has on fecal ingredients which may cause development of cancer (these are referred to as carcinogens) and the faster passage of stool through the bowel, thereby reducing contact time and cell damage (see further discussion in chapter 9). It is estimated that in some countries of Africa the incidence of colon cancer is less than five cases per hundred thousand people, while in parts of the United States the incidence is higher than thirty cases per hundred thousand people. In Senegal, for example, the incidence rate is 1.9 cases per hundred thousand population.

In further support of the connection of diet to colon cancer are a number of "migrant studies" which have examined the incidence of the disease in ethnic groups who have emigrated to other countries which have a contrasting rate of colon cancer occurrence. For example, studies of Japanese immigrants to the United States showed that the mortality rate of colon cancer among males rose to the prevailing rate or higher than the one among Caucasians. Similar results were found in Chinese and Polish immigrants to the United States and in Polish and southeast Asians who emigrated from their native countries to Australia. Ethnic groups who emigrate and maintain their native cuisine are likely to have colon cancer incidence rates closer to those in their native country, as was reported in another study that looked at southern Europeans (especially Greeks and Italians) who emigrated to Australia. Thus, change of diet appears to be an important factor in change of incidence of colon cancer. On the other hand, all immigrants to the United States do not necessarily acquire the same risk of colorectal cancer shown by native-born Americans. Examples include Mexicans (who have half the rate of colorectal cancer than native-born white Americans do) and Puerto Ricans. In most studies, the rates of colorectal cancer in immigrants to the United States rose more in males than in females.

Overeating, weight gain in adulthood, and obesity are strongly implicated as risk factors for colorectal cancer. In one California study, investigators found that not only were obesity and weight gain associated with the presence of adenomatous polyps, but so was weight variability over a ten-year period. Additionally, sedentary lifestyle or occupation poses a risk for colon cancer. People who have high levels of physical activity have a reduced risk of developing colorectal cancer; even simple activities such as regular walking have been found to be beneficial in protecting women from developing colon polyps.

Studies have suggested that dietary calcium plays a role in protecting against colon cancer; it may do so by binding fatty acids and bile acids and directly inhibiting abnormal growth of colon epithelial cells. Likewise, some studies have shown that colon cancer rates in areas that have high groundwater and soil concentrations of the element potassium may have lower rates of colon cancer. Of interest is the finding of lower colon cancer rates in people with Addison disease, Parkinson disease, and schizophrenia, all of which are conditions associated with higher cell concentrations of potassium. Higher rates have been reported in conditions associated with low cell concentrations of potassium such as obesity, alcoholism, Crohn disease, and Cushing disease.

Recent research suggests that persons who supplement their diet with at least eight hundred micrograms of the vitamin folic acid on a daily basis have a reduced incidence of colon cancer. There is also evidence that aspirin and related drugs may reduce colon polyp development and colon cancer incidence. These findings have provoked great interest and further research into the causes and possible prevention of colon cancer, particularly the cellular mechanisms by which colon cancer develops and the means by which these drugs may reduce the development of colorectal cancer (see chapter 9).

Therefore, it is postulated that materials in the diet that are carcinogenic or converted to carcinogens in the colon act to disturb the glandular cells of the colon and are the cause of cancer-promoting mutations (gene mutations). Fat is strongly suspected to be an important promoter of colon carcinogenesis.

Socioeconomic, Religious, and Ethnic Factors

Colon cancer rates appear to be somewhat influenced by economics, regional geography, religion, and social stratification. For example, the highest rates of colon cancer in the United States occur in the Northeast, and lower rates are seen in the South. Rates are higher in urban areas than in rural areas. One suggested explanation of this urban-rural difference is that rural people have more exposure to the sun, with subsequent increases in vitamin D production and calcium absorption (see chapter 9). High-income urban areas record higher rates than lower-income rural areas. In the United States, Caucasians and blacks have higher rates of colon cancer than do Hispanic Americans or Native Americans. Ashkenazi Jews have higher colorectal cancer rates than the general population in both the United States and Europe. In Hawaii, the male:female incidence ratios are highest in the Japanese and Chinese residents of the islands. But the incidence of colon cancer in the United States is much lower in Mormons and Seventh-Day Adventists (religious groups which eschew smoking and alcohol and practice forms of dietary moderation) and vegetarians. California Seventh-Day Adventists (about half of whom are lacto-ovovegatarians) appear to have mortality from colorectal cancer that is almost one-half that of white males of comparable socioeconomic status. Mormons do not have a diet that is particularly low in fat but do favor balanced diets containing fruits, vegetables, whole grains, and modest amounts of meat. In other words, Mormons have a fairly typical American diet but place more emphasis on whole grains and fiber-containing foods than other Americans do. Their colon cancer incidence is a little under two-thirds of the average incidence for white males in the United States. Yet the complete story for why there is a reduced risk of colorectal cancer in Mormons and Adventists remains to be clarified.

The Polyp-to-Cancer Sequence

While the biochemical and genetic mechanisms of colon carcinogenesis may still be incompletely understood, it is well established that the anatomic precursor of colon cancer is the adenomatous polyp. (A polyp is a growth protruding from a mucous membrane. An adenoma is a benign growth from a glandular tissue, such as the mucous cells lining the intestine.) People who have adenomatous polyps in the colon are at increased risk of developing cancer.

The evidence for the sequence from polyp to cancer is from studies that have shown that people who have had polypectomy (removal of polyps) and are followed up with removal of any subsequent polyps have a significant reduction in the incidence of colon cancer. Removal of premalignant polyps stops the progression from adenoma to adenocarcinoma, and can save lives.

If a polyp is found, the likelihood that it is cancerous is increased if the polyp is large and if it is adenomatous (glandular). Nonadenomatous polyps are not considered to be precancerous. The finding of only nonadenomatous polyps on a screening examination does not predict a higher likelihood of adenomatous polyps. If a polyp is larger than two centimeters in diameter, there is a 50 percent probability that it will contain cancerous cells. Adenomatous polyps may be tubular, villous, or tubulovillous. Villous polyps are characterized by finger-like projections and are about ten times more likely to contain cancer cells than tubular adenomatous polyps. Tubular polyps are closely packed and rounded in appearance. Tubulovillous polyps are intermediate between tubular and villous. It is believed that a large (more than one centimeter) adenomatous polyp takes about five and a half years to transform into a cancer. Polyps in the left colon have a statistically lower chance of harboring cancer than polyps in the right colon.

Polyps may be sporadic (meaning that they occur in a random or unpredictable manner) or may occur in well-defined inheritable syndromes. These are described below. But it is important to remember that sporadic polyps are a very common finding in all people.

The Polyposis Syndromes

Several inherited syndromes are characterized by polyposis and increased risk of colon cancer.

Familial adenomatous polyposis (FAP) is the most important of these syndromes, yet it accounts for less than 1 percent of colon cancers in the United States. Affected individuals develop hundreds or thousands of polyps by their teen years, any one of which may develop into a cancer. Eighty percent of individuals with FAP will also develop small bowel adenomas, and 50 percent will develop polyps in the stomach. There is increased risk of cancer of the first portion of the small bowel (duodenum), and in Japanese people there is increased risk of cancer of the stomach. Two-thirds of individuals with FAP will also develop a condition in the eye known

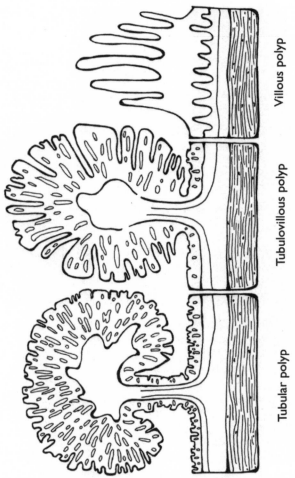

FIG. 1.1. Schematic representation of tubular, villous and tubulovillous polyps.

as congenital hypertrophy of the retinal pigment epithelium (CHRPE). CHRPE does not affect vision, nor does it have a malignant character, but it is an important marker of the FAP syndrome and can be detected at birth by ophthalmologic examination. CHRPE is best described in plain English as freckles on the retina (the portion of the eyeball that receives images and transmits visual impulses to the brain).

FAP has an autosomal dominant pattern of inheritance. Autosomal means that the gene is not on a sex chromosome, so its inheritance is not sex-related (as is the hemophilia gene, for instance, which is on the X-chromosome and so can be passed to males only from their mothers). Either the father or the mother can pass along the FAP gene, and the disorder can occur in males or females with equal likelihood. Dominant means that only one gene is needed to produce the effect. Based upon prevalence of FAP in the general population, it is estimated that the gene is present in one in every five thousand to seventy-five hundred persons.

Preventive action, usually consisting of repeated examination or removal of the colon, is necessary, along with careful screening of family members for this disorder. The APC (adenomatous polyposis coli) gene, located on human chromosome 5, is believed to be the responsible gene for FAP.

Gardner syndrome is probably a variant of FAP; it occurs about half as frequently and has similar clinical features, such as CHRPE. It may affect the small intestine as well as the colon. Benign tumors affecting bone (osteomas), connective tissue (fibromas), fatty tissues (lipomas), the tissues lining the abdomen (desmoid tumors), and benign cysts of the sweat glands (sebaceous cysts) may be found.

Oldfield and Turcot syndromes might be related to FAP. The former is associated with sebaceous cysts. The latter is associated with tumors of the central nervous system and may be transmitted by an autosomal recessive gene (recessive means that for the condition to be expressed, a copy of

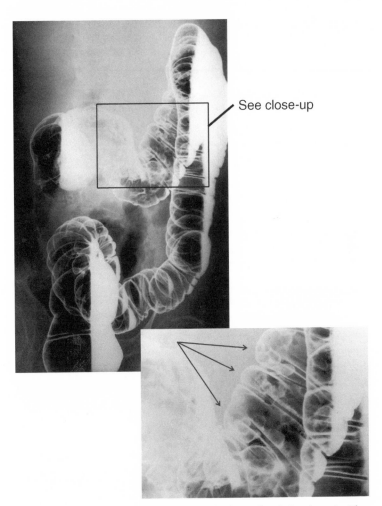

See close-up

FIG. 1.2. Barium enema and close-up which shows familial polyposis. The polyps are outlined by the white silhouette of barium on the x-ray. This individual had Gardner's syndrome and underwent colon removal (total colectomy) at the age of thirty-five. Later, he developed massive desmoid tumors. This patient's mother, brother, and son all had Gardner's syndrome.

the gene must be inherited from each parent). Studies have differed on the finding of APC gene mutations in Turcot's syndrome. Both syndromes are quite rare.

Hereditary nonpolyposis colorectal cancer (HNPCC) has a name that is somewhat misleading, because these forms of colon cancer do in fact arise from polyps, but individuals do not have an abundant proliferation of polyps as in the above-mentioned polyposis syndromes. The polyps that are found in family members have an extraordinarily high likelihood of progressing to cancer. Therefore, it is felt that these individuals have a cancer gene more than a polyp gene. That is, they may be as likely or only somewhat more likely than the rest of the population to develop polyps, but once these polyps arise, such persons are genetically predisposed to have cancer develop in one of them at a much higher rate than are others with polyps.

The syndrome of family clustering of colon cancer was first recognized in 1913 by Alfred Warthin. HNPCC is also known as the Lynch syndrome, named for Dr. Henry Lynch, a pioneer researcher in the field of cancer genetics who followed up on the original family studied by Warthin and studied other families as well. There are two Lynch syndromes: Lynch I, in which only colon cancer is passed along, and Lynch II, in which both colon and noncolon cancers (especially ovarian and uterine) are inherited.

HNPCC accounts for about 5 percent of colon cancer cases. The incidence of this syndrome has been controversial, because until recently there has been little objective means of identifying people with it. Criteria for inclusion of cases into this syndrome were published by the International Collaborative Group on Hereditary Nonpolyposis Colorectal Cancer. These three criteria are referred to as the Amsterdam Criteria.

Individuals with HNPCC have a strong family history of colon cancer (Lynch I) and sometimes other forms of cancer as well (Lynch II). Colon cancer in individuals with

Table 1.1. The Amsterdam Criteria for Hereditary Nonpolyposis Colorectal Cancer

---

1. At least three relatives have colon cancer with at least one being a relative in the immediate family
2. Two successive generations must be affected
3. At least one individual must be diagnosed before the age of 50

HNPCC looks just like sporadic cases of colon cancer, but the polyps that lead to colon cancer have a much more aggressive and malignant nature. Often multiple colon cancers are found, either at the same time or at different times in a person's life.

Determining that a person has this form of colon cancer necessitates taking a careful family history to establish the genetic nature of the disorder. This obviously also has important implications for the children of a person with the disorder. The polyps found in individuals with this hereditary condition are thought to have a greater and more rapid potential for becoming malignant than those found in persons without the disorder.

Screening of family members of patients with this disorder should start at an earlier age than screening in the general population and should be done more frequently.

Risk of colorectal cancer in the families of patients with nonhereditary adenomatous polyps was examined in the National Polyp Study when 1031 patients with adenomatous polyps were interviewed about their family history. The risk of colon cancer in their siblings or parents was almost twice that expected, and was almost three times the rate expected when the polyps were discovered before a person reached the age of sixty.

Sporadic Colon Cancer Cases

The majority of colon cancer cases (at least 85 percent) are thought to be sporadic in nature. These occur in individuals with no identifiable hereditary disorder that predisposes them to colon cancer, and are likely initiated by environmental carcinogens alluded to above leading to a series of accumulated genetic alterations or mutations which result in a malignant tumor. These types of mutations are called somatic mutations, meaning that they occur not in the germ cells of an organism but in the cells of body tissues.

These somatic mutations lead to overproliferation of mucosal cells of the colon, which then lead to aberrant crypt foci that can become adenomas or polyps. Most polyps do not become cancerous. As will be seen below, a series of additional somatic mutations is required before cancer develops. The complete sequence of mutations may take up to ten or twenty years before cancer develops (see chapter 3).

Inflammatory Bowel Diseases

People with inflammatory bowel diseases are at increased risk of colon cancer. These include ulcerative colitis and, to a lesser extent, Crohn disease. (See *Understanding Crohn Disease and Ulcerative Colitis* by Jon Zonderman and Ronald S. Vender, M.D.)

Ulcerative colitis is a chronic disease of the large bowel that has episodic behavior and an unpredictable outcome. It is characterized by recurrent inflammation and ulceration of the colon and rectum and primarily involves the innermost layer of the colon, called the mucosa (see chapter 2). The etiology, or cause, of this disease is unknown. Clinically, the prominent symptoms of ulcerative colitis are diarrhea and bleeding. Other symptoms of attacks are abdominal pain, fever, and weight loss. The risk of colon cancer from ulcerative colitis increases when the entire large bowel is involved and also increases with the length of time a person has been known to have had the disease. Since ulcerative colitis is a lifetime disease, the risk of colorectal cancer is higher in people who are first diagnosed with ulcerative colitis at a young age (especially if they are under twenty-five). The average age for diagnosis of colorectal cancer in patients with ulcerative colitis is forty-nine years, compared to sixty-nine years in the general population. Additionally, cancers tend to be multifocal (that is, multiple cancers at different sites in the large bowel) about 40 percent of the time. Cancer usually occurs in parts of the bowel that are inflamed by the disease process itself, but can also occur in areas of the bowel not involved by ulceration. Prevention of colon cancer usually entails resection (removal) of the entire large bowel.

Crohn disease is likewise a chronic and episodic disorder of the bowel, but can affect the entire gastrointestinal tract from mouth to anus. It is distinguished from ulcerative colitis by its involvement of the entire wall of the bowel, not just the mucosa. It is usually most prominent in the small bowel, colon, and anus. The risk of colon cancer from Crohn disease is less than that from ulcerative colitis, but may be as high as twenty times the expected incidence in the general population. The average age of cancer occurrence is forty-eight years.

Other Risk Factors

People who have had previous colon cancer, breast cancer, ovarian cancer, and endometrial cancer are at risk of having cancer of the large bowel. A history of radiation to the pelvis for other cancers such as cervical, bladder, and endometrial seems to raise the risk of colon cancer, too.

Schistosomiasis, a parasite that occurs primarily in Africa and Asia, may increase colon cancer risk, although data to support this is scanty. Schistosomiasis is caused by any of several species of parasite flatworms of the genus *Schistosoma*, which affect about two hundred million people worldwide.

There have been some studies of both humans and mice that suggest that cholecystectomy (gallbladder removal) may increase a person's odds of having colon cancer. Other studies have contradicted these findings. Nevertheless, it is an intriguing concept, given that removal of the gallbladder alters the patterns of metabolism of bile, which may be a factor in colon carcinogenesis.

Ureterosigmoidostomy (creation of a connection of the ureter via the sigmoid colon to the outside of the abdomen) may lead to cancer at the line of connection between the ureter and the colon. It is thought that a urinary ingredient is converted to a carcinogen when exposed to the bacteria of the bowel.

Occupational exposure probably does not play a major role in the development of colon cancer, although isolated reports of clusters of colon cancer in people of various occupations have been made. Those in occupations that have been implicated include brewery workers, crystal glass foundry workers, automobile model and pattern makers, and workers exposed to formaldehyde.

2. The Colon

The large intestine comprises the appendix, cecum, colon, rectum, and anal canal. The colon comprises the ascending colon, transverse colon, descending colon, and sigmoid colon. The colon wall contains four layers of tissue: the mucosa, submucosa, muscle layer, and serous layer.

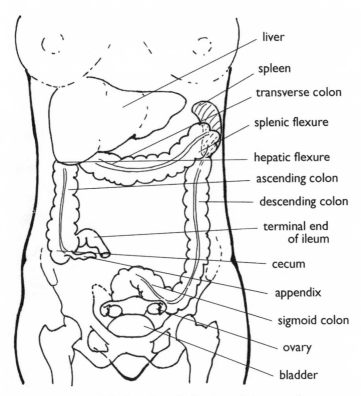

FIG. 2.1. Anatomy of the large bowel, showing relations to other anatomic structures and circulation.

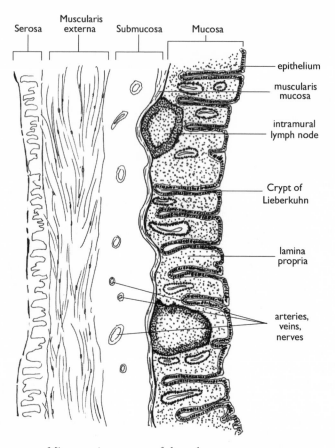

FIG. 2.2. Microscopic anatomy of the colon.

It is the epithelium of the mucosal surface that is exposed to fecal carcinogens, and it is there that the vast majority of colon cancers begin. Colon epithelium has a flat surface and contains many long, thin tubular glands known as crypts. (They are sometimes also called the glands of Lieberkühn after the eighteenth-century German anatomist who first described them.) The crypts measure about half a centimeter in depth (0.2 inches). The deeper portion undergoes constant cell division so that the epithelium is replaced completely every four to six days. Because dividing cells are vulnerable to genetic damage, the epithelium is particularly sensitive to noxious substances. (It is because of the constant turnover and sensitivity of gastrointestinal epithelium that nausea, vomiting, and diarrhea are common side effects of chemotherapy drug and radiation therapy; see chapter 8.)

The colon mucosa contains absorptive cells that absorb water and electrolytes and goblet cells that produce mucus. There are at least a dozen and a half or more different types of cells, which secrete hormone-like peptides into the adjacent lamina propria and into the lumen of the bowel. These peptides have a variety of functions important to digestion and the motility or propulsive action of the colon.

The lamina propria is a mesh of tissue primarily containing collagen (a type of connective tissue) that occupies the space between crypts in the epithelium and the muscularis mucosa. Interestingly, it also contains lymphocytes and other cells of the immune system (called mast cells, plasma cells, macrophages, eosinophils, and fibroblasts). The exact role and function of these cells is not clear. Blood and lymph vessels, as well as nerve fibers, are found here.

The thin muscularis mucosa is situated at the base of the lamina propria and is spread like a sheet of fine filo dough.

Blood Supply of the Colon

The vascular system of the colon includes arteries, which deliver blood rich in oxygen and nutrients, and veins, which carry oxygen-poor blood to the lungs and heart. Surgical decisions regarding resection of colon cancers depend heavily on their location in the colon and on the blood supply to that particular segment. The chief arterial sources are the superior mesenteric artery and the inferior mesenteric artery, which branch off the aorta, the very large artery that comes directly from the heart. The superior mesenteric artery through its branches provides blood to the small bowel, right colon, and transverse colon. These branches are the ileocolic artery, which supplies the cecum, appendix, and final portion of the ileum; the right colic artery, which supplies the right colon; and the middle colic artery, which feeds the transverse colon. The inferior mesenteric artery through the left colic artery branch feeds the left colon and through the sigmoidal arteries and the hemorrhoidal arteries supplies the rectum. Each artery has a complementary vein with a corresponding name.

The Lymphatic System

Lymphatics are vessels that drain the fluid known as lymph from tissues and return it to circulation. Lymph consists primarily of lymphocytes and fluid containing fat and protein. Lymphoid cells are interspersed throughout the tissues of the colon, while lymph nodes are found in networks adjacent to or just outside of its walls. Lymph nodes are part of the immune system and are important in the defense against invasion by viruses, bacteria, and cancer cells. Hundreds of lymph nodes are present in all parts of the body, and lymphocytes, like an army of microscopic FBI agents, provide biological surveillance against the anarchy that can result from infection and malignancy.

Colon lymph is drained to three main groups of lymph nodes: the paracolic nodes, which essentially border the outside surface of the colon; the intermediate nodes, which skirt along the major arteries supplying the colon; and the central nodes, which are rooted near the aorta. The lymph drains through this network of nodes and eventually finds its way into a large sac (or reservoir) of fluid known as the cysterna chyli, which then drains into another large vessel, the thoracic duct. The thoracic duct flows into the left subclavian vein, which carries blood and lymph into the vena cava, from whence they are recycled into the arterial side of circulation through the heart.

The lymphatic network of the colon plays an important role in both inflammatory bowel disorders and cancer.

Physiology and Function of the Colon

The chief functions of the colon are the formation and temporary storage of stool. The colon is not essential to life—since people can survive after its removal—but the study of people who have had their large bowel removed sheds light on its important functions. Lack of a colon leads to the following conditions: (1) excessive loss of sodium and chloride ions and water, (2) chronic dehydration and low sodium levels in the blood, and (3) a compensatory decreased urine production by the kidneys. The latter situation may lead to increased production of kidney stones.

Bacteria play an important role in colon physiology since it is through their fermentation action on undigested fiber and residues that production of short-chain fatty acids depends. It is estimated that four hundred bacterial species take up residence in the large intestine, and it is believed that this diversity is due to the large number of available energy sources; each species may have evolved a special niche in terms of energy ecology. The bacterial population in the colon is influenced by diet, age, and geographic location of the host. Short-chain fatty acids may be a significant energy source useful in body metabolism. Additionally, colonic bacteria help convert urea, a waste product, into ammonia which can be reabsorbed and metabolized. Uric acid and creatinine are other products of metabolism that can be metabolized further by the action of fecal bacteria. The human colon therefore has a small but not insignificant nutritive role in human physiology through the action of bacteria on fiber and subsequent production of short-chain fatty acids. The colon is also capable of absorbing simple substances such as sugars, amino acids, and fatty acids that may play a role in human nutrition.

Bacteria may also play an important role in colon carcinogenesis (see chapter 3). Bacteria may break down bile acids into carcinogens. The mutagen fecapentaene is produced by members of the bacterial genus *Bacteroides*, which is found in the colon. Dietary constituents may have a role in inducing colonic bacteria enzymes that may either promote or retard carcinogenesis.

As mentioned above, the colonic epithelium produces a number of hormones (enteric peptides), most of which regulate bowel action. Small amounts of hormones with activity in other parts of the body are thought to be produced by the colon as well.

Clinical Correlations of Anatomy to Colon Cancer

Because of the relatively larger capacity of the cecum and right colon, cancers located there may have a more insidious growth and development. The larger caliber of the cecum and greater degree of elasticity permit cancers to grow to a larger size before being felt or diagnosed.

On the other hand, cancer of the left colon tends to make itself felt sooner than right-sided lesions. Because of the relatively smaller caliber and greater firmness of the descending colon, tumors there are more likely to cause constriction and obstruction.

3. How Colon Cancer Develops

Carcinogenesis is the process by which cancer is produced. Carcinogenesis is caused by genetic damage to cells. It is *not* an infectious process. (Note: certain infectious diseases that are transmissible from person to person may create conditions that permit cancer to develop, but the cancer cells themselves are not infectious.)

Genetic material is contained in the cell nucleus. It consists of deoxyribonucleic acid, or DNA. DNA is involved in the reproduction of the cell and how it functions (that is, what type of organ it will be part of and what it will do in that organ) and determines most of the attributes of the living organism. The cell is bounded by a membrane, which serves as a site of receptors for hormones and proteins from other cells that may send signals to the cell. The membrane, by virtue of the physical barrier that it creates and the receptor molecules that are located on it, also serves as a gatekeeper that keeps out or permits molecules to enter the cell cytoplasm.

All cancers begin with cells that have accumulated genetic changes, or mutations, which cause the cells to lose normal control of reproduction and differentiation (maturation to their specific individual form and function). These abnormal cells produce progeny that have the same mutations. The majority of colon cancers are the result of either inherited genetic abnormalities that predispose a person to cancer or the accumulation of cancer-producing mutations under the steady influence of environmental stresses. We will be discussing these pathways to cancer in further detail below.

Cancer is a disease of uncontrolled cell reproduction and loss of differentiation. Current theory holds that carcinogenesis is due to cells losing through a series of mutations the ability to regulate cell death. These immortal cells have lost the ability to undergo the genetically programmed process known as apoptosis, which permits a cell to complete its natural life cycle. Cancerous cells may therefore both proliferate and accumulate. Cells that are relatively old are prone to accumulate further genetic damage from exposure to genotoxins such as drugs and radiation. Cells may therefore be susceptible to further instability and malignancy. The immortal cells of cancer, much like vampires, eventually kill the organism that feeds them.

Carcinogenesis is a slow process. Cancer does not develop in a matter of hours or days or even weeks. Multiple phases are involved in carcinogenesis that may take years or even decades to evolve. The steps in colon carcinogenesis beginning with a normal cell and ending with a clinically apparent cancer may be summarized as follows:

1. *Initiation.* In this phase a normal cell is "initiated" into the path towards malignancy by a mutation.
2. *Clonal expansion.* The cells do not yet appear neoplastic (cancerous), but have accumulated as clones which make them ready to take the next step toward cancer. In colon carcinogenesis, this may appear as aberrant crypt foci in the mucosal epithelium.
3. *Benign tumor formation.* Further genetic changes have turned a preneoplastic clone into a benign neoplasm (tumor). In colon cancer, this is the polyp phase (also known as adenoma or adenomatous polyp).
4. *Malignant tumor.* Further mutations in the cells of an adenomatous polyp have converted it to a malignant tumor.
5. *Clinical cancer.* The malignant tumor has now acquired the properties of what is clinically referred to as cancer: the tendencies to invade and to metastasize (spread).

Research suggests that the average time of progression from initiated cell to adenomatous polyp is five years. The same amount of time is probably required for an adenomatous polyp to become invasive cancer. The long amount of time between adenoma and cancer provides the rationale for colon cancer screening. If polyps are detected early, the progression to cancer can be stopped.

Certain individuals are genetically predisposed to develop colon cancer. Such individuals have a colon composed entirely of cells which already are "initiated." Sporadic colon cancer, on the other hand, requires the cumulative acquisition of mutations in colonic mucosal cells that result in cancer formation. The accumulation of these mutations requires the influence of environmental (mostly dietary) factors. The risk of occurrence of such an accumulation of mutations in the general American public is estimated to be about 5 percent.

When someone speaks of colon cancer, it is understood that the specific category of cancer being referred to is an adenocarcinoma. This type of cancer arises from the mucosa of the large bowel. While benign and malignant tumors can arise from other cell types such as muscle (known as leiomyomas and leiomyosarcomas) and lymphocytes (lymphomas), these are quite rare. Adenocarcinoma refers to the glandular nature of the cells and tissue from which it derives. (Adenos is the Greek word for gland; carcinoma refers to an epithelial malignancy.)

The Molecular Genetics of Colon Cancer

Although FAP and HNPCC account for only a small percentage of all colon cancer cases, the mutations identified in those disorders help provide an understanding of the mutations which occur in sporadic colon cancer. There are two defined molecular pathways that lead to colon cancer, the chromosomal instability pathway and the hypermutability, or microsatellite instability, pathway. Each step in the pathway endows the cells with a greater degree of instability, which eventually leads to actual malignant transformation.

The Chromosomal Instability Pathway

The chromosomal instability pathway accounts for probably 85 percent of sporadic cases of colon cancer. In this pathway, the cancer sequence begins with a mutation in the APC (adenomatous polyposis coli) gene. This gene is located on chromosome 5, has been implicated in FAP, and is a tumor suppressor gene. Tumor suppressor genes block uncontrolled cell proliferation. Damage or loss of a tumor suppressor gene is analogous to losing the brakes in a car. Once there is loss of function of this gene, there is a loss of normal cell mortality, and cells proliferate abnormally. The normal function of the APC gene is not known but the hypothesis is that it plays a role in maintaining cell structure. Damage to the APC gene may result in the formation of an adenoma which is chromosomally unstable (hence the name of this pathway) and a propensity to lose entire chromosome segments, which results in further genetic loss and instability.

Furthermore, mutation of the APC gene may lead to activation of an oncogene called c-MYC. Oncogenes are analogous to gas pedals in a car. They turn on or promote the process of carcinogenesis. APC also interacts with a cellular protein called beta-catenin, responsible for keeping normal cells stuck together in an orderly array. Therefore loss of APC gene function reduces normal cell-to-cell adhesiveness and predisposes to random and disorderly cell growth.

Loss of APC may be necessary, but is not sufficient to cause cancer. The next step down the path to cancer may be misfunction of a gene known as K-ras located on chromosome 12. K-ras is a protooncogene, that is, a gene that can, after mutation, become an oncogene, or tumor promoter.

Oncogenes are involved in signal transduction, so that continued promotion of tumor growth occurs. Mutation of the K-ras gene has been likened to a situation in which the accelerator is stuck to the floor. Without the APC gene mutation, however, K-ras does not cause cancer. If APC is intact, K-ras by itself will result only in a condition known as aberrant crypt foci.

The third gene mutation in this pathway to colon cancer development is likely a mutation of another tumor suppressor gene known as DCC (for "deleted in colorectal cancer") or possible other gene located on chromosome 18. DCC may be part of a larger cluster of genes that are part of the pathway to cancer. In one study, patients with colon cancer with an intact DCC had a much higher survival rate than those without intact DCC; thus, identification of DCC mutation may serve as a prognostic indicator.

The fourth step in this pathway is the disabling of the p53 gene, a tumor suppressor gene that is important in suppressing a number of cancers besides colon cancer. At least 50 percent of colorectal cancers have an inactivated p53 gene. This gene is located on chromosome 17; it appears to be involved in recognizing that DNA damage has occurred and keeps the cell from replicating. If genetic repair cannot be performed, p53 probably stimulates apoptosis. Thus, loss of p53 permits abnormal cells to avoid death and continue to proliferate without restraint.

The Microsatellite Instability Pathway

This pathway is implicated in HNPCC and about 15 percent of sporadic cases of colon cancer. Throughout its lifetime, a cell may be exposed to mutagens. In colon cancer, at least some of these mutagens may be in the stool that passes over the bowel mucosa and may damage its DNA.

DNA is a very long molecule that is composed of double helical strands connected to each other like rungs of a ladder by molecular fragments known as nucleotide bases. The four nucleotide bases are adenine, thymine, guanine, and cytosine. These four bases form the genetic code. In normal DNA, adenine pairs only with thymine, and guanine pairs only with cytosine. However, mutagens can cause mistakes in the way nucleotide bases pair, and this is referred to as DNA mismatch.

Normally the cell responds to DNA mismatch by means of mismatch repair. Disturbances of the DNA mismatch repair system (MMR) can result in a situation known as microsatellite instability. Microsatellite instability refers to abnormal variations in short, repetitive DNA sequences.

Five different mismatch repair genes have been identified: MSH2, MLH1, PMS1, PMS2, and HMS46. Fifty percent of families with HNPCC have mutations of MSH2, and 30 percent have a defect in MLH1. Mutations of the other three genes, PMS1, PMS2, and HMS46, are rare.

Mutations in the MMR system may be necessary but are not sufficient to result in cancer. Other mutations must occur in the pathway to malignancy. The defect in DNA repair genes leads necessarily to mutations in other genes, including tumor suppressor genes and oncogenes, which lead to tumor development. Colorectal cancers with microsatellite instability tend to have a more favorable prognosis (the forecast of probable outcome of the disease), but the reason or reasons for this are not at all clear.

It was recently reported that people who have deficiency of the enzyme alpha-1-antitrypsin (important in lung and liver function) have a threefold increased risk of developing a microsatellite "instable" colon cancer, and this risk increases in smokers.

Sporadic Colorectal Cancer

A multistep model for colorectal carcinogenesis has been proposed:

1. Colorectal cancers are clonal (meaning they develop from a single cell) and arise as the result of mutations which activate oncogenes and/or inactivate tumor suppressor genes.
2. Several genes (sometimes as many as four or five) must be mutated to cause cancer.
3. These gene mutations do not have to occur in any specific order. Only the total accumulation of the mutations matters.
4. Dysfunction of both copies of a gene is not always necessary to produce cancer.

4. The "Look" of Colon Cancer

The Signs of Colon Cancer and Tests Used by Physicians to Diagnose It

A "symptom" is an abnormality felt by a person. A "sign" is an abnormality observed by a physician or other health care professional in a physical examination or in a laboratory or x-ray examination. Symptoms are the "feel" of a disease or disorder and will be discussed in chapter 5. Signs are the "look" of a medical problem.

The Physical Examination

When someone with colorectal cancer in the early stages walks into a doctor's office for an examination, the most likely circumstance is that neither the patient nor the physician will feel or see an obvious sign of cancer. Yet finding cancer in its earliest stages, when a patient is asymptomatic, provides the greatest opportunity for cure.

The most important test for colorectal cancer that a physician performs during a physical examination is the digital rectal exam (DRE). After taking a good look at the anus to see if there are abnormalities such as hemorrhoids, warts, fissures, fistulas (abnormal opening to the external surface), skin tags or tumors prolapsing (protruding) from the rectum, the physician performs a careful finger examination. Wearing latex gloves, the examiner inserts the index finger through the anus and into the rectum. Lesions in the rectum up to seven centimeters (2.75 inches) from the external boundary of the anus can be detected with the sweep of the finger. It is estimated that this examination can detect as many as 15 percent of colorectal cancers.

The DRE can give a wealth of other information to the physician. In addition to palpating the sacrum and coccyx (the tailbone structures) and some of the muscles of the pelvic floor and the anal sphincter, the examiner will be able to feel the prostate and seminal vesicles in men and the cervix and other structures of the female pelvis in women. Tumors of these other organs may be felt during the exam, and gentle pushing with the finger against the rectal tissues in different directions may detect tenderness caused by inflammation of the peritoneum (the membrane that lines the abdominal cavity and encloses the abdominal organs).

After performing the digital examination, the examiner wipes some stool from the examining glove onto a filter paper containing a peroxide-sensitive chromogen (or color chemical indicator) and then places drops of a developing solution containing hydrogen peroxide on it. If any amount of the enzyme peroxidase is present, it causes the hydrogen peroxide to break down to water and oxygen. Oxygen produced in this reaction in turn causes the chromogen to turn blue. Thus, blood or hemoglobin (which has peroxidase activity) in the stool will undergo a chemical reaction with the hydrogen peroxide to yield oxygen that further reacts with the chromogen to leave a blue color. The presence of blue color indicates that there is bleeding somewhere in the gastrointestinal tract. This is called the fecal occult blood test (FOBT) and is an important part of screening tests for colorectal cancer. Certain vegetables that have peroxidase activity and hemoglobin from undigested meat can give a false positive reaction. Vitamin C and other agents that interfere with the peroxide-peroxidase reaction will give a false negative reading. The FOBT is sometimes referred to as the stool guaiac, a throwback to the days when a resin from trees of the genus Guajacum (found in the Dominican Republic and Haiti) was used as the chromogenic material on the filter paper.

Examination of the abdomen may reveal a mass if the cancer is much enlarged. If the cancer is causing obstruction, there may be distention of the abdomen with gas causing a drum-like sound when the abdomen is tapped. Bowel sounds may be high-pitched if there is an obstruction. Tenderness, another possible sign of colon cancer, may be elicited by the examiner when the abdomen is tapped upon or palpated. Enlargement of the liver may be felt if there has been spread of the cancer to the liver. This may be detected as hard nodules dispersed in the liver or as a general fullness in the right upper portion of the abdomen, where the liver is located.

In the early stages of colorectal cancer, the physical examination may be entirely negative. For this reason, other screening techniques for early detection of colorectal cancer are advised.

Anemia

Because colorectal cancer may cause bleeding, anemia is a frequent sign. When viewed with a microscope, the red blood cells (RBC) appear pale and small due to lack of hemoglobin which is caused by iron deficiency. Bleeding removes iron, a major component of red blood cells, from the body.

In adult women who are menstruating and/or have recently borne children, iron deficiency anemia is a common finding. Childbirth contributes to iron deficiency in women by several mechanisms: (1) the increase in the maternal blood volume which develops in pregnancy results in consumption of stored iron in the body tissues, (2) blood loss can be a consequence of bleeding which may occur at the time of delivery, and (3) diversion of maternal iron stores to the developing fetus depletes the mother of her iron.

Although it can be found in young children whose dietary intake of iron is outstripped by their growth or in adults who are severely nutritionally deprived or are unable to absorb dietary iron, iron deficiency in otherwise normal American adults is in almost all cases due to internal bleeding from the gastrointestinal tract.

Bleeding from the gastrointestinal tract can occur from ulcers, varicose veins in the esophagus or stomach (usually due to chronic liver disease), stomach irritation (gastritis), aspirin use, hemorrhoids, polyps, blood vessel malformations, diverticulosis, colitis, and cancers. When iron deficiency anemia is found in a man or in a woman who is not actively menstruating or who has not borne several children, a thorough examination of the bowels is required to prove that cancer is not the cause.

In iron deficiency anemia, automated blood analyzers will show that the mean corpuscular volume (MCV)—or size—of the red blood cells is smaller than normal (less than 82 cubic microns). The value in normal individuals should be between 82 and 101. The level of iron in the blood (serum iron) is low, the iron-binding capacity (the availability of storage sites on iron-carrying proteins) is high, and the transferrin saturation is low. (Transferrin is a protein that facilitates transport of iron in the blood.) A particularly good test for iron deficiency is the serum ferritin level. Ferritin is a protein that facilitates storage of iron. When the blood ferritin level is abnormally low, there is a good chance of iron deficiency. Blood cells are made in bone marrow, and in cases where there is doubt about the cause of anemia, it may be necessary to perform a bone marrow biopsy to prove that the cause is lack of iron. Bone marrow can be examined and treated with chemical stains to reveal whether there is iron present or not. Absence of detectable iron in the bone marrow is a reliable indication that the person has iron deficiency.

In more advanced stages of colon cancer, anemia may be a result of the effects that chronic illness or treatment have had on the patient. Liver function impairment and malnutrition are factors that have a role in causing anemia. The type of anemia seen under these circumstances is called normocytic anemia (red blood cell size is normal). Chemotherapy drugs may cause normocytic or macrocytic anemia (red blood cells are of large size) by suppressing the normal production of red blood cells by the bone marrow. In such situations, the use of recombinant human erythropoietin (Procrit) to stimulate red blood cell production may be of value (see chapter 8).

Other Blood Tests

Tumor markers are substances found in blood, tissues, and bodily fluids that are associated with cancer activity. These are usually proteins which are uniquely expressed (or produced) by cancers and not by normal tissues. These tests are not used as screening tests because of the unacceptable incidence of false negative and positive results that may occur, but are used when a cancer diagnosis has been established by other means. Their chief application is for monitoring response to therapy.

The identification of tumor markers results from the search for immunologic differences between normal and cancerous cells. The term "immunologic" refers to the presence of unique proteins on cells (antigens) against which antibodies can be formed. These antibodies can be labeled and used as identifying tags on the tumor marker protein. Normally these antigenic proteins are expressed only in the embryological stages of human development. They may be detected, however, in tumor cells that have reverted to a more primitive or embryological stage.

The major tumor marker for colorectal cancer is CEA, which stands for carcinoembryonic antigen. This was first discovered in 1965 in fetal intestine, liver, and pancreas and in cancerous adult liver, colon, and pancreas. CEA may be identified in cancer cells by special staining techniques and may be measured in the blood. Such stains for CEA may be used by pathologists to distinguish normal from cancerous tissue and in an effort to determine the organ of origin of an adenocarcinoma. Because elevated CEA levels are found in cancers besides colorectal, they are not diagnostic for colorectal cancer. The normal blood level of CEA is 0–5 nanograms per milliliter. But serum CEA concentration is an extremely useful tool for monitoring the results of therapy, and a decreasing serum concentration of CEA following colon cancer treatment is an indicator of effective treatment, while a rising concentration is an indicator of increasing cancer activity. Rising CEA concentration may precede other clinical symptoms of colorectal cancer activity and may be an indication for further investigation. In some cases where the CEA is rising, a "second-look" operation may be performed. CEA may have some prognostic value, since a preoperative level greater than 10 ng/ml suggests that the cancer is already metastatic (has spread to other organs). The more advanced the colon cancer, the more likely it is that CEA will be elevated.

Even when cancer is advanced or widespread, CEA is not always elevated. Reports have shown that 60 to 94 percent of patients with recurrent or metastatic colorectal cancer will have an elevation of CEA. Similarly, elevated CEA does not always mean cancer. Benign conditions which may cause an elevated CEA test are hepatitis, liver injury from anesthetics, gallbladder and bile duct inflammation, bowel inflammation, and cigarette smoking. Thus, CEA must always be interpreted with caution and by someone who is knowledgeable and experienced in its interpretation.

Other tumor markers for colorectal cancer include CA 19–9, CA 196, TAG 72, and CA 50. Of these, only CA 19–9 has been used much in clinical settings. No tumor marker has been used as frequently as has CEA for colorectal cancer.

X-rays and Other Imaging Studies

Plain x-rays are the type that is taken when a person has, for example, a routine chest x-ray. A plain x-ray is a study in contrasts between the appearance of gas-density material (like air), the appearance of water-density tissues (also referred to as soft tissue), and the appearance of mineral densities like bone. Plain x-rays of the abdomen are frequently not useful for the diagnosis of colorectal cancer because the appearance is usually normal. However, indirect signs of cancer may be seen and may lead the physician to suspect cancer when symptoms are present. It is rare that a colorectal cancer is of sufficient size that it can be seen as a soft tissue mass on a plain x-ray, but the occasional case does arise when a mass, silhouetted by bowel gas, can be distinguished by a skilled radiologist. A more typical finding on a plain x-ray in the presence of colon cancer is a normal pattern of gas, but if the cancer is causing obstruction, there may be distention and dilation of the bowel with large amounts of gas. If the cancer is in the rectum and is causing obstruction, there may be a sudden disappearance of gas immediately beyond the obstruction. If a cancer has caused perforation of the colon, free gas may be found as a bubble underneath the diaphragm.

When colon cancer has spread to the lungs, a chest x-ray may show nodules that are indicative of metastases.

The traditional way of diagnosing large bowel lesions for many years was by means of the barium enema. This test is preceded by a careful cleansing of the bowel to permit the introduction of barium into the colon and rectum. Barium is an inert material that is radiopaque, meaning that x-rays cannot penetrate through it, and light or white areas are left on x-ray film wherever it lies. Preservatives and other materials are mixed with the barium and help it give a cast, or outline, of the bowel mucosa. Growths such as polyps and cancers will have a typical appearance.

There are various methods by which barium enemas can be performed. The single contrast examination involves the filling of the colon with a continuous column of barium under pressure through a tube placed just past the anus. Lesions in the lumen of the colon will leave darker areas (called filling defects) which may have a diagnostic or characteristic appearance. In order to get the best possible views and avoid overlapping of images, film exposures are taken with the patient in multiple positions. Postevacuation films (taken after the barium has been expelled) are helpful in getting better

Table 4.1. A Sample Method of Preparation for Flexible Sigmoidoscopy or Barium Enema

Day 1	
All day	Clear liquid diet. Examples: clear bouillon, apple juice, cranberry juice, plain Jell-O
3 P.M.	Drink one bottle of citrate of magnesia
Day 2	
All day	Clear liquid diet
Early A.M. (on rising)	Use a Dulcolax suppository
1 P.M.–6 P.M.	Drink an 8-ounce glass of water every hour
2 P.M.–3 P.M.	Take 2 ounces of castor oil or repeat citrate of magnesia
Day 3	
Day of exam	Nothing by mouth until the exam is completed

views of filling defects in the bowel and in distinguishing true defects from stool which may have been retained.

To get the most accurate impression from a barium enema, double contrast (sometimes called air contrast) is used. That is, both barium and air are inserted into the colon so that a thin layer of barium outlines the mucosa while the lumen is filled with air. Again, the most optimal study is obtained when the patient is x-rayed in multiple positions.

The technique of double contrast barium enemas was developed after flexible fiberoptic colonoscopy (see below) became available and showed that a significant number of colon lesions were being missed by single contrast enemas. When properly performed and interpreted, the double contrast barium enema is superior to the single contrast barium enema for diagnosis of colon cancer and polyps, especially when the lesion is smaller than two centimeters in diameter. The use of single contrast is preferred only if the patient is too old or feeble for air contrast, has extensive diverticulosis, or has had prior removal of the ileocecal valve.

Sometimes a biphasic examination—one in which a single contrast (barium only) enema is followed by a double contrast examination—may be necessary when the findings of the single contrast study are inconclusive. This may occur when fecal material is seen sticking to the bowel wall and if it is questionable whether there truly is a growth or not. If the ileocecal valve is open during the test, it may be easy to miss a malignant growth.

Distinguishuing between a benign polyp and a small malignant one may be difficult. If the outline of the growth is irregular or has a broad base or seems to cause pinching or narrowing at that particular point, it is more likely to be a malignant growth. Rapid growth of a polyp between two different barium enema examinations points to it being malignant.

Larger growths tend to encircle the bowel lumen and invade further into the bowel wall. This may give the edges of the lesion a shelf-like appearance. Encircling of the bowel may give the cancer an annular, or ring-like, appearance. "Apple-core" and "napkin-ring" lesions are terms used by radiologists to characterize such a tumor cast.

In some cases of colon cancer, the barium enema may reveal a stricture. This is a long narrowing of the bowel that may be caused by cancer spreading under the mucosal surface. Malignant strictures can also be caused by long-standing ulcerative colitis. Radiation therapy, ischemic colitis, granulomatous colitis, and ulcerative colitis may cause benign strictures.

Barium enemas may reveal obstruction, perforation, fistula formation, intussusception (collapse of one part of the colon into another part), and ischemia (diminished blood supply), all of which are potential complications of colon cancer.

Double contrast barium enemas have a 70 percent or better detection rate of polyps that are larger than seven millimeters (approximately a quarter of an inch). For colorectal cancer, detection rates are variable, according to different studies which have been performed to answer the question of how reliable barium enemas are in ruling out cancer. The results have ranged from a low of 70 percent reliability to a high of 96 percent.

Complications of barium enemas are few. The most serious complication is perforation of the wall of the colon. The incidence of perforation ranges from 0.1 to 0.01 percent of tests performed. Perforation may be caused by direct damage from the enema tip or from increased pressure on the bowel wall caused by the column of barium or by the air that is used in a double contrast study. Perforation may be complicated by peritonitis (inflammation of the abdominal cavity), which can be life threatening or fatal. Impaction (blockage) with barium can occur, especially if there is an area of narrowing in front of the column of barium. Dehydration and hypoglycemia can occur, especially in the elderly or in those with diabetes. Water overload is a rare complication that may occur, particularly in kidney dialysis patients.

Cat Scans

Computerized axial tomography (CAT) is a technique in which computers are used to reconstruct detailed representations of internal anatomy. Cross-sectional x-ray images of the body are obtained when an x-ray tube and detectors rotate around the patient. The technique has been so refined over the last twenty years that excellent detailed pictures can be obtained in twenty minutes or less. The main advantages of CAT scans are that internal organs, blood vessels, lymph nodes, and nerves can be distinguished in much better detail than in plain x-rays. In addition, images of the internal organs can be obtained in any of the three-dimensional projections, since the cross-sectional images can easily be reformatted by the computer.

CAT scans may not reveal direct evidence of a bowel cancer or polyps, since currently used techniques in community practice do not permit reliable evaluation of lesions in the bowel lumen. Therefore, CAT scans are not presently used in screening for or diagnosis of colorectal cancer. (This may change in the future, however, as "virtual colonoscopy" becomes further developed for community use; see chapter 10.) However, CAT scans may show indirect evidence highly suggestive of cancer in the bowel or evidence of spread of cancer to other internal organs.

For example, CAT scans may show thickening or stricture of the bowel wall that may indicate the presence of a malignant lesion. Perforation of the bowel caused by cancer may also be seen along with formation of an abscess near the perforation site. Bowel obstruction may be seen and is characterized by dilated loops of bowel proximal to (ahead of) the obstruction. Abnormal soft tissue density in the abdomen or pelvis may be an indication of a colon or rectal cancer that has penetrated the wall of the bowel and is invading local tissues.

Evidence of metastasis to the liver is seen when there are filling defects of the liver on a CAT scan. Metastasis to the lungs may be seen with the spots that appear abnormally on the scan.

Ultrasound

Another type of imaging is provided by ultrasound. Ultrasound is identical to sonar: it is a technique of sending out and then detecting sound waves which bounce off internal organs (known as echogenicity). From ultrasound it can be determined if the liver has homogeneous density of its tissues. Metastases may appear as characteristic changes of the normal homogeneic echogenicity of the liver. If an advanced colon cancer has caused blockage of the bile system, ultrasound may be helpful in demonstrating this problem.

Endoluminal (rectal) ultrasonography is of particular use-fulness for rectal cancers. In this procedure, a probe is placed into the rectum and sound waves are produced from the lumen of the rectum, giving a close-up and accurate ap-praisal of the rectal tissue. This technique can help determine thickness and penetration of a rectal cancer and may help determine if nearby lymph nodes are involved.

Nuclear Medicine

Technetium-99 liver-spleen scans. The inert and harmless radioisotope of the element technetium is injected into the bloodstream to obtain an image of the liver. Although this scan has been a helpful test for decades, its use as a diagnos-tic test in colon cancer is limited to the detection of metas-tases to the liver. Although this test provides remarkably good accuracy and is relatively cheap, it has been largely replaced by CAT scans for determination of cancer spread.

Nuclear scintigraphy. Scintigraphy involves the use of ra-diolabeled antibodies to detect the tumor marker CEA. A number of such antibodies have been developed, but clinical usefulness and reliability of these tests have been uneven. The ideal clinical application of such a test would be to localize cancer if the blood CEA level is high but other imaging techniques fail to show signs of cancer. One study has shown that scintigraphy alone or in combination with CAT scanning provided better preoperative assessment of patients than CAT alone.

PET scans. In positron emission tomography (PET), as in other nuclear medicine scans such as the technetium-99 liver-spleen scan, a radioactively tagged (but completely harmless) compound is injected into a patient to obtain internal images of the human body. However, a major distinction of PET scanning is that it can shed light on metabolic activity of tumors. PET scanning has been around for approximately as long as CAT scans (about twenty-five years) but has been relegated until recently to being a research tool in academic centers. However, PET scanning appears to be gaining acceptance by insurers as a cost-effective and superior technique of cancer imaging, and is now entering the mainstream as a diagnostic tool in the community at large. A positron is a positively charged electron that passes through a few millimeters of tissue before it collides with a negatively charged electron, thereby creating two photons (particles with momentum and energy). These two photons are emitted in opposite directions and are detected simultaneously as "coincident" photons. A PET scanner has a ring of detectors surrounding the body which localize the positron-electron "annihilation" events which occur, and, depending on the type of positron-emitting material used, can detect various metabolic functions of body tissues and organs. Most PET scanning techniques rely upon the fact that cancer tissues consume increased quantities of glucose as an energy source and therefore utilize a positron-labeled form of glucose to identify cancers and metastases as "hot spots" on a scan. In many cases, the metabolic activity of cancers which can be detected by PET technology precedes the anatomic changes which are detectable by CAT scans or other modalities. In one study, PET scans were found to be more accurate than CAT in detecting colorectal metastases both inside and outside the liver. Thus PET scans may be of great help when cancer activity is suspected but not localized by other diagnostic tests.

MRI

Magnetic resonance imaging (MRI) has limited usefulness for establishing if visceral organ metastases are present, since it is more expensive but probably no better than CAT scans.

However, MRI may be of help in cases where the CAT scan findings are equivocal. It is also useful in the diagnosis and evaluation of rectal cancers. As MRI machines with shorter image times are developed, this technique may take on a more prominent role in the future for imaging of cancer.

Endoscopy

The development of fiberoptics has ushered in a whole new approach to the diagnosis and treatment of colorectal cancers. In no other organ of the body except the esophagus and stomach is it as possible to examine the entire "field" for cancer as it is in the colon. The inner portion of this hollow tube, the mucosa, is where 90 percent or more of colon cancers begin. Flexible scopes which can be navigated through the bends, twists, and gyrations of the large bowel make it possible to directly scrutinize the inner cavity where malignant and premalignant changes can be identified.

Anoscopy uses a simple rigid metallic or plastic speculum (opening device) to examine the anus. It is readily available in most doctors' offices and requires no preparation. For patients with bleeding, itching, pain, tenesmus, narrowed stools, and other symptoms, anoscopy may give immediate information such as the presence of hemorrhoids. This test should not be performed if a patient has pain or narrowing of the anus.

Rigid sigmoidoscopy is a procedure that has fallen out of fashion because of the availability of flexible scopes. However, there are still indications for use of the rigid proctosigmoidoscope, which unfortunately has acquired a bad image owing to the discomfort that the procedure may cause. The rigid scope permits a more thorough and accurate exam of the rectum, especially when the examiner is looking for a cause of bleeding, and is sometimes used before barium enema and colonoscopy. Rigid sigmoidoscopy can be performed with less preparation than other techniques.

Flexible fiberoptic sigmoidoscopy (also referred to more casually as "flex sig") is used to examine only the left colon, rectum, and anal canal. This procedure can be performed by primary care physicians, internists, surgeons, and gastroenterologists to screen and diagnose large bowel disorders, including polyps and cancer. These scopes have a diameter between one and one and a half centimeters. Various conditions that may prompt a physician to recommend this procedure include family history of polyps or colon cancer, bloody stool, diarrhea, abdominal or rectal discomfort, and change of bowel habits. Sigmoidoscopy should not be performed if a patient has had a recent heart attack or recent pelvic or rectal surgery and should not be performed if there exists an indication to perform a full colonoscopy.

Flex sigs are performed in a doctor's office or in dedicated endoscopy suites of a hospital or outpatient surgery center. A careful preparation is required, which can be similar to the one performed for a barium enema. The patient lies on the left side on an examining table or gurney, curled up in the fetal posture with buttock pointing outward toward the examiner. The physician may have an assistant to help guide and propel the scope. Before insertion of the scope, a visual examination of the anus is performed, followed by digital (finger) examination of the rectum. The scope is then inserted and gradually pushed to the target distance (which varies from thirty-five to seventy centimeters). Flexible endoscopes are equipped with an air line so that air can be inflated into the bowel to help open it up. As the examination proceeds, the physician follows the lumen with the scope to eventually reach the target distance. The examination can reach as far as the splenic flexure if required. Since flex sigs are not customarily performed with the assistance of sedation, these examinations may be limited or cut short by the discomfort sometimes brought on by these exams.

Colonoscopy, which is the extension of flexible fiberoptic endoscopy for examination of the entire large bowel, eliminates some of the guesswork that is sometimes evoked by barium enemas and flex sigs. Colonoscopies are performed by gastroenterologists (physicians who specialize in diagnosis and treatment of disorders of the digestive system) and surgeons (general surgeons as well as those specializing in colorectal diseases).

Colonoscopy, like barium enemas, requires a careful cleansing and catharsis of the bowel to permit a clean view of its inner anatomy. Often, this is given as a one- or two-day preparation in which the individual undergoing the test takes a potent cathartic (such as GoLYTELY) to eliminate all stool. Unfortunately, the volume of GoLYTELY required to cleanse the bowel is large (four liters). The taste of GoLYTELY is rather disagreeable; getting the last drop down can be a forbidding and formidable task. The test is performed in an outpatient endoscopy center and requires conscious sedation, usually with the help of a drug called Versed and other medications to prevent pain, nausea, and bowel spasm. This drug has the capacity to make a person very drowsy and relaxed but not fully anesthetized or unconscious. The patient is carefully monitored during this procedure so that abnormal lowering of blood pressure and pulse will be avoided.

Colonoscopy is beginning to supplant flex sig as the preferred endoscopic method of bowel examination. It is a more reliable test and may be more cost effective as a screening method for colon cancer than other tests. Factors limiting its use are restrictions raised by insurance companies and managed care, limited availability of the test due to limited availability of trained physicians, expense, inconvenience, and the more ready availability of other tests such as barium enema and flex sig. (There may be more physicians in communities who are trained to perform flex sigs than there are specialists who can perform colonoscopy.) Colonoscopy should be performed in patients with prior history of colon cancer, personal or family history of polyps, and when there is blood in the stool. Other indications may include changes in bowel habits, abnormality seen on barium enema, and unexplained diarrhea and abdominal pain. Since hemorrhoids are so common, the finding of hemorrhoids on other examinations should not be taken at first blush as the only explanation for a person's bleeding. If a polyp is found on a flex sig, then colonoscopy should be advised so that the rest of the colon can be examined for more polyps.

Modern endoscopy equipment permits viewing of the procedure on a video monitor as it is performed, and photographs of areas of interest or abnormality can be obtained on the spot. Colonoscopes are equipped with water and suction apparatus so that cleanup can be done as needed during the procedure. Wire loops, snares, and forceps useful for performing biopsies or excisions of suspicious growths are available.

Colonoscopy has a detection rate of at least 85 percent of colon cancers. In one study, the detection rate was 95 percent when the test was performed by a gastroenterologist and 87 percent when it was performed by nongastroenterologists. Colonoscopy is superior to barium enema for detection of polyps and other lesions smaller than half a centimeter, but it is questionable whether lesions this small have great clinical significance. Colonoscopy should not be performed if a person has had a recent heart attack, stroke, or abdominal surgery.

Intraoperative colonoscopy is the use of colonoscopy during surgery, while a patient is under anesthesia, to ensure complete and thorough examination of the large bowel. Studies have shown that the use of intraoperative colonoscopy may result in the finding of a significant number of synchronous (coincident) polyps and early cancers at the time of surgery for a previously diagnosed cancer.

Pathologic Appearance of Colon Cancer

The gross appearance—that which is visible to the naked eye—of colorectal carcinoma is usually either that of a polypoid lesion (protruding growth) or of an annular constricting lesion. Polyps may have a rounded appearance with no stalk

**Table 4.2. Side Effects and Potential Complications
of Endoscopy**

- The bowel preparation may lead to dehydration, mineral and electrolyte imbalance, and, in the infirm, could lead to pneumonia and congestive heart failure.
- Gas-like discomfort or cramping is likely to be felt during the procedure. Since air is used to inflate the bowel, the urge to pass gas may be experienced. The instrument itself may create the sensation of having to move the bowel. This is normal and can be helped by expelling the gas.
- Pain of a sharp nature is not normal and should be reported immediately to the physician who is doing the procedure.
- Bleeding may result if a biopsy is performed or if the scope traverses a fragile area of tissue.
- Spasm of the bowel may occur, which may make passage of the colonoscope difficult or more uncomfortable.
- Perforation of the bowel is possible, but unlikely to occur if an experienced endoscopist performs the procedure. Infection or bleeding could complicate perforation, and hospitalization could be required.

(these are referred to as sessile) or may appear as a stalk and bud (pedunculated polyps). Polypoid lesions tend to be more common in the right colon (where there is more distensibility of the bowel and more room for growth), while the ring-like annular constricting lesions are more common in the left colon. As the cancer grows, it may develop into a large, irregular, and expansive fleshy mass on the lumen of the large bowel. It may or may not show ulceration and bleeding, and it may show nearby satellite growths. A flat, diffuse, infiltrating type of cancer (one which spreads across the superficial layer of the bowel lumen) is more common in patients who have had ulcerative colitis.

The microscopic pathology of colorectal cancers will show a proliferation of cells in an uncontrolled and random manner in later stages. In the earliest stage, when still confined to a polyp, it may show as an in situ (in place) carcinoma. The vast majority of colorectal cancers are adenocarcinomas, meaning that they are of glandular origin. Therefore, a rudimentary appearance of gland-like structures may be seen under the microscope. Occasionally, cells will take on a signet-ring appearance, owing to the presence of large globules of mucus-like material within the cell cytoplasm.

Cancerous cells may be seen dividing and invading into blood vessels and lymph vessels within the wall of the bowel itself. The pathologist will report findings such as this, and will be most interested in determining the depth of invasion of the cancer into the deeper layers and surrounding tissues of the bowel wall. The pathologist will also describe how well differentiated (that is, how close to mature, normal cells and cell arrangement) the cancer is and how aggressive its behavior appears to be. About 20 percent of colorectal cancers are described as "poorly differentiated." The less well differentiated a carcinoma is, the higher its grade (aggressiveness and tendency to invade and spread) is felt to be. While grading of colorectal cancers has some usefulness from the clinical standpoint, the partially subjective nature of tumor grading makes it difficult to achieve uniformity from one hospital or medical center to another, and it is therefore less useful as a comparative prognostic feature. Of great significance is whether there is invasion of lymph nodes, as this is the most important prognostic factor in colorectal cancer. (Invasion of lymph nodes by cancer is indicative of beginning stages of cancer metastasis.)

A metastatic adenocarcinoma discovered in another part of the body and suspected to be originating from the colon may be tested with special stains to determine the primary site of origin. One such stain is the CEA stain, which, when positive, may suggest bowel origin of the cancer.

5. The "Feel" of Colon Cancer

Symptoms of Colon Cancer

Perhaps the most common occurrence in the early stages of colon cancer is that the individual feels nothing. This is the best time to find and cure colon cancer and is the reason that screening examinations are promoted by so many leading medical organizations. Solid scientific data clearly supports the notion that early detection of colon cancer can be life saving. It is the same principle applied to the use of mammography and Pap smears for detection of breast cancer and uterine cancer.

Bleeding

The symptom most often associated with colon cancer is blood in the stool. Occasionally a person first notices blood on toilet paper after wiping. This may be ignored or passed off as hemorrhoidal bleeding. However, blood in the stool is sometimes a difficult thing to sense. Bleeding may occur so slightly that it is not visible to the naked eye. The normal brown color of the stool masks small volumes of blood, and the fact that bleeding has occurred may only be detected through tests. Black stool may also be caused by the ingestion of iron supplements or bismuth preparations (such as Pepto-Bismol).

Blood in the stool is the consequence of bleeding from an ulcerating lesion in the gastrointestinal tract. Ulcers in the stomach and duodenum, for example, are a common cause of bleeding in the upper portion of the gastrointestinal tract. In the colon and rectum, bleeding may occur from several different possible causes. Perhaps the most common cause is hemorrhoids. Another common source of blood in the stool is diverticulosis, a condition in which small out-pouchings are found in the wall of the colon, especially the descending portion. Abnormal blood vessel formations may also cause bleeding. Superficial blood vessels in bowel mucosa may be abnormally dilated and prone to break open and bleed in these conditions. Anal fissures may also bleed.

However, the most ominous causes of bleeding are polyps and cancers of the colon. Therefore, any time blood is found in the stool by patient or physician, it must be taken as a serious matter. The cause must be determined. Blood in the stools, no matter what the cause, is not normal.

It is not unusual for people to be unaware of the fact that bleeding is occurring. When the bleeding is too slight to be visible, it may be detected by the fecal occult blood test (see chapter 4).

Constant bleeding may lead to anemia, a condition in which there is a deficiency of hemoglobin or red blood cells. The hemoglobin in red blood cells carries oxygen to cells, enabling them to carry out metabolism and growth. In particular, muscle tissues (including the muscular tissue of the heart) are very greedy consumers of oxygen. Therefore, when a person becomes anemic, common feelings in the early stages are fatigue that comes easily or lack of stamina. As anemia becomes worse, a person may become noticeably pale and may experience breathlessness and rapid pulse with minimal exertion.

The character of the blood in stool is dependent upon the location in the large intestine where bleeding occurs. The higher up in the bowel, the darker the blood's appearance. Thus, blood from a right-sided colon lesion will give a darker red (brick-colored) appearance. Bleeding from the left colon may commingle with stool to give it a brown-red appearance, while rectal bleeding will cause the stool to be coated with the bright red appearance of fresh, untouched blood.

Changes in Bowel Habits

If a colon cancer is a constricting lesion, that is, one that causes the bowel to narrow down and choke the passage of stool through it, a person may notice that the stools have a narrower caliber. This is more likely to occur in cancers involving the left portion, since stool is still predominantly in liquid form in the right colon and cecum. The smaller caliber is sometimes referred to as "pencil-thin" stools. Other alterations of bowel habits may occur, including diarrhea, constipation, or the complete inability to have a bowel movement, known as obstipation, a symptom very suggestive of bowel obstruction. Bowel obstruction is a dangerous complication of colon cancer and is considered a surgical emergency. Other signs of large bowel obstruction include abdominal distention, bloated feeling, and pain. Diarrhea is frequently seen in certain types of polyps known as villous adenomas. These polyps are spongy, leafy growths that tend to spread out and can cause a person's bowel habits to change from normal to a very watery diarrhea. Villous adenomas frequently contain small focal points of malignant cells. Occasional patients may present with alternating constipation and diarrhea that may mimic the irritable bowel syndrome. Cancers of the rectum frequently present with a change in bowel habits, particularly increased frequency.

Abdominal Discomfort

Lower abdominal pain, bloating, and cramping are some of the symptoms of colon cancer. When symptomatic, right-sided colon lesions are likely to cause a vague ache. This discomfort may become more defined and localized to the right side of the abdomen as the cancer grows. An examining physician may feel a palpable mass in the right side. If the cancer causes a perforation of the bowel, the abdominal pain may simulate the pain of appendicitis or that of a gallbladder attack.

Left-sided colon lesions tend to give colicky discomfort. This is a bit of a redundancy, since the word "colic" actually refers to the colon. However, as generally used, "colicky" means a fluctuating, deep visceral discomfort brought on by contractions of the bowel wall muscle during peristalsis.

Particularly long, painful, and ineffective straining at defecation, known in medical terms as tenesmus, may be another symptom, particularly of rectal cancers that are causing obstruction. Fullness in the rectum, pressure, and incomplete evacuation of stool are other symptoms of rectal cancers. Pain, not an early sign of rectal cancer, may occur as a result of direct growth by the cancer into the adjacent organs such as bladder, vagina, uterus, or ureters, or it may be caused by the spread of cancer cells along nerves. Pain in other parts of the body may be indicative of cancer that has spread to other organs, such as the liver.

Occasionally rectal cancers close to the anus may cause prolapse (or protrusion of rectal tissue) out of the anus, which the person may feel. An unusual symptom is passage of stool through the urine caused by a fistula into the bladder resulting from a colorectal cancer which has grown into the bladder. In women, a similar situation may occur into the vagina, resulting in passage of stool via that orifice.

Phlebitis and Pulmonary Embolism

For reasons not completely understood, most cancers, including colorectal cancer, have a proclivity to enhance blood clotting, a situation that can have potentially serious complications. The fine balance that normally exists between the fluid nature of blood and the congealed state that is needed if tissue is cut is somehow tilted in favor of clotting in cancer patients. Typically, blood clots begin in the deep veins of the calves and thighs and result in phlebitis (swelling, warmth, redness, and discomfort). If a piece of the blood clot breaks off and migrates in veins back to the heart, it could eventually lodge in one of the vessels feeding the lungs and result in the choking off of oxygen to lung tissue and death of the tissue, causing shortness of breath and chest pain or in the patient's death.

Shingles

Shingles is a painful skin eruption that is caused by reactivation of the chicken pox virus herpes zoster. The occurrence of shingles may be a random event, but it is also believed that shingles may result from a disruption of the immune system that permits the attack to take place. Such immune system disruptions may occur before, during, or after the diagnosis of colorectal cancer (and other cancers) has been made.

Signs of Advanced Disease

The early stages of colon cancer may display fairly specific and localized symptoms as described above. If cancers spread to other organs, symptoms that may follow include general effects such as weight loss, weakness, malaise, loss of appetite, and fever. Organ-specific symptoms occur according to the affected organ. The organs most likely to be affected are the liver and lung.

If cancer has spread to the liver, pain localized to the right upper portion of the abdomen may be felt. This pain may be caused by the stretching of the liver capsule brought about by enlargement of the liver due to tumor metastases. Pain may also radiate to the back or to the shoulder.

If cancerous cells massively replace the normal liver tissue, the organ's function is impaired and jaundice develops. Jaundice is caused by circulating bilirubin, a breakdown product of hemoglobin. The yellow pigment accumulates in the skin and the eyes. Jaundice can also result from blockage of the bile ducts outside of the liver, if cancer cells have spread to that location.

The liver is an important site of blood protein production, so if the liver is failing in its function, a state of malnutrition and a low blood concentration of albumin ensues. Albumin is the major protein in blood and is responsible for a number of important functions, including transport of ingested drugs and important blood constituents such as hormones. Albumin is also responsible for preventing fluid to leak out of blood capillaries by the process of osmosis. Thus a lower than normal concentration of albumin may result in fluid retention in, for example, the abdominal cavity or the feet and ankles. Sometimes the state of protein malnutrition is so severe that fluid collects around the lungs and causes severe shortness of breath. Fever may also be caused by cancer metastases to the liver, since cancer cells are capable of releasing fever-causing chemicals.

A state of near complete liver failure may cause coagulation disturbances and bleeding due to inability to synthesize blood-clotting factors. (The liver is the site of production of most blood proteins, including clotting factors.) The liver is also important as a site of production, storage, and release of glycogen. Glycogen is a large complex molecule composed of units of glucose (a sugar used by the body for immediate energy needs). Liver failure may therefore also result in severe hypoglycemia due to inability to produce glycogen. Coma may be the final result of overwhelming liver failure brought on by cancer.

When colon cancer has spread to the lungs, symptoms may be absent at first or may later be quite noticeable. A simple cough may be the first sign. Later, as the size and number of lung metastases increases, there may be increasing cough, sometimes of a bloody nature, as well as shortness of breath, chest discomfort and tightness.

Occasionally advanced colon cancer cases may spread to the lining of the abdominal cavity, the peritoneum, and may result in fluid leakage into the abdominal cavity. This may be another way in which ascites (see above) is caused. Abdominal distention and bloating may result. Encroachment of cancer on loops of small bowel and large bowel may cause further pain, bloating, and bowel obstruction.

6. Stages and Prognosis of Colon Cancer

Staging of cancer is the essential step in the process of determining both treatment and prognosis. It is a fundamental part of any cancer treatment plan, for without an accurate determination of the stage of a person's cancer, it is not possible to make a sensible conclusion about which treatment should be employed.

The same type of cancer may have quite contrasting treatment plans and prognoses if the stages are different. The use of certain approaches for individuals whose colon cancer is confined to the mucosa and of others for people whose cancer has already spread to the liver is probably easily understood even by those who have no medical knowledge or training. In one situation, aggressive therapy, primarily consisting of surgery, is readily applied, with the expectation that the individual should be cured of the disease. In the other, surgery would likely *not* be a consideration. "The tumor was inoperable"—an assertion loaded with dramatic innuendo of prognostic significance—is perhaps the most concise yet easily appreciated statement of cancer staging.

Current staging systems of colorectal cancer stem from earlier versions initially used for rectal cancer. Even the early systems recognized the fundamental importance of the following features in determining less favorable prognostic aspects: (1) depth of penetration beyond the mucosa, especially the importance of penetration of the muscularis propria or extension to fatty tissue outside of the colon, (2) involvement of lymph nodes, and (3) overall size of the tumor.

The Dukes Classification

Cuthbert Dukes was a London pathologist who published in 1932 a modified staging system of rectal cancers in which he set apart three stages, A, B, and C, and was able to correlate five-year survival with the staging system. Stage A included carcinomas confined to the wall of the rectum. Cancers that spread into the tissues immediately outside of the rectum but did not involve lymph nodes were included in stage B. If lymph nodes were involved, then the cancer was stage C.

Dukes's original system for rectal cancers was modified by other investigators for use in staging *all* colorectal cancers.

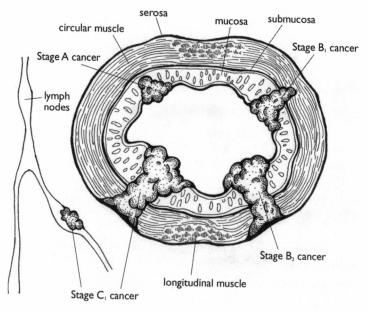

FIG. 6.1. Schematic representation of the different stages of colon cancer, according to depth of penetration into the bowel wall and involvement of the nearby lymph nodes.

The staging system used today for colon and rectal cancers is commonly referred to as the Astler-Coller modification of the Dukes classification system. The modern version of this modification adds a stage D, which includes patients whose tumors have spread to other organs.

The TNM Staging System

Over the course of time, various staging systems involving both alphabetical and numeric grades have evolved for different cancers. In an effort to give systematic uniformity to cancer staging, the tumor-node-metastasis, or TNM, system was published in 1954 and was later adopted by the American Joint Committee for Cancer Staging and End Results Reporting.

In this system of staging, classification is built upon three criteria: the size or extent of the primary tumor ("T"), status of involvement of the lymph nodes ("N"), and presence or absence of metastases to organs or sites distant from the origin ("M"). Metastasis refers to the process of cancer cells escaping from their site of origin and spreading, either via the

Table 6.1. The Astler-Coller Modification of the Dukes Staging System[*]

Stage A: Tumor involving the mucosa only
Stage B_1: Tumor within the wall; nodes are negative
Stage B_2: Extension through the wall; nodes are negative
Stage C_1: Tumor within the wall; regional nodes are positive
Stage C_2: Extension through the wall; regional nodes are positive
Stage D: Distant metastatic disease

---

*Other modifications of the basic Dukes system of staging exist

bloodstream or the lymphatics, to other organs. Metastases or metastatic lesions are tumors that have secondarily implanted and grown in other organs or tissues different from the primary site. Thus, a colon cancer that has spread to the liver and lungs has metastasized to these organs.

A numeric stage is then determined from the three components given above.

The following examples may help the reader understand this system better (these are true clinical cases, although the names have been changed).

Example 1. Mr. Miles Coltrane, a seventy-five-year-old jazz musician, was seen for an annual physical and was found to have anemia. He had virtually no other complaints, but when questioned a little he did mention an intermittent vague abdominal discomfort that he attributed to "indigestion." Investigation of the anemia revealed that it was due to internal bleeding and that the bleeding was coming from a tumor in the cecum which was visible on a barium enema. He underwent colonoscopy by a gastroenterologist, and biopsy of the lesion revealed that he had adenocarcinoma. He was then operated upon by a surgeon who removed the cecal mass and the ascending colon. The surgeon also looked at the liver and saw no obvious sign of cancer involvement. The pathologist who examined the tissue that was removed reported that the cancer penetrated into the muscularis propria but did not involve any lymph nodes or adjacent fatty tissue. The cancer was staged an Astler-Coller B_1, or stage I ($T_2N_0M_0$) according to the AJCC Group Staging Criteria. Mr. Coltrane did not require any further treatment.

Example 2. Ms. Ruby Bright was about to go on a shopping spree to New York. She had just celebrated her twenty-fifth anniversary. The night before her departure, she experienced a frightening episode of fresh blood in her stool. She immediately called her internist, who performed a sigmoidoscopy examination the next morning. Expecting to find only hemorrhoids, the doctor was surprised to discover a

Table 6.2. The TNM and Group Staging Criteria for Colorectal Cancer with Astler-Coller Equivalent

T_1 Involves the submucosa but does not invade the muscularis propria

T_2 Invades but does not penetrate the muscularis propria

T_3 Penetrates through the muscularis propria; may penetrate into the serosa (if present) or pericolic fat, but not into the free peritoneal cavity, nor does it invade other organs

T_4 Invades other organs or involves the free peritoneal cavity

N_0 No nodal metastases

N_1 One to three pericolic (directly neighboring the colon) or perirectal (directly neighboring the rectum) nodes involved

N_2 Four or more pericolic or perirectal nodes involved

N_3 Involvement of any regional node along a blood vessel

M_0 No distant metastases

M_1 Distant metastases present

AJCC Group Staging Criteria		Astler-Coller Equivalent
Stage I	$T_1N_0M_0$	A
	$T_2N_0M_0$	B_1
Stage II	$T_3N_0M_0$	B_2
	$T_4N_0M_0$	B_2
Stage III	$T_{1-2}N_{1-3}M_0$	C_1
	$T_3N_{1-3}M_0$	C_2
	$T_4N_{1-3}M_0$	C_2
Stage IV	$T_{any}N_{any}M_1$	D

large bleeding tumor that was about thirty centimeters from the anus. A CAT scan of the abdomen did not reveal any suspicious lesions in the liver. The surgeon then performed a sigmoid colon resection. Pathology disclosed that the cancer penetrated completely through the bowel wall and involved the adjacent pericolic fat. Seven lymph nodes were seen in the resected specimen, and none of them had cancer. The cancer was therefore stage Astler-Coller B_2, or stage II ($T_3N_0M_0$) by the AJCC system. After a consultation with a medical oncologist, it was decided that Ms. Bright should undergo adjuvant chemotherapy.

Example 3. Mrs. Polly Posis saw her doctor every year on the day after her birthday for a physical. It had been over five years since her last flexible sigmoidoscopy, and the doctor recommended that the procedure be performed again. A polyp was found in the rectum, fifteen centimeters from the anus. This was removed and a tiny cancer was found at the base of the polyp. She had a low anterior resection of the rectum. Pathology showed that it had not yet gone into the muscularis propria layer. Her cancer was eventually staged $T_1N_0M_0$ (stage I), or stage A according to the Astler-Coller system.

Example 4. Dr. Rollo Tomasi, a fifty-four-year-old pharmaceutical chemist, sought the medical advice of his family physician when he developed an itch around the anus. His grandson had just been treated for pinworm, and he suspected that he had acquired the same problem. (Normally he did not like to see doctors.) His doctor did not see much of anything around the anus and did not feel a mass or hemorrhoids during the rectal examination. The doctor, who doubted that Dr. Tomasi had pinworm, thought it might be a good idea to do a flexible sigmoidoscopy. To everyone's amazement, a large polypoid mass was found about fifty centimeters from the anal verge that to the naked eye had all the features of a cancer. The biopsy revealed an adenocarcinoma. Dr. Tomasi subsequently had an operation to remove the sigmoid colon, and, while exploring the rest of the abdomen, the surgeon found three suspicious nodules in the liver that also proved to contain adenocarcinoma. Because five lymph nodes were found to be positive, the cancer was staged $T_3N_2M_1$ (stage IV, or Astler-Coller D).

Prognosis

Factors that Affect Prognosis

Age. A young age may portend a worse prognosis, but how much worse is difficult to measure. The fact that colon cancer is much less common in people under the age of forty than in older people makes getting statistically valid comparisons difficult in the study of survival rates. Cancers in younger people tend to be more poorly differentiated (more aggressive in nature), and more of these individuals have Dukes C stage (this could be because the level of suspicion regarding young people is low, which allows the cancer to escape earlier detection). Old age in itself is not a negative characteristic unless the patient has cardiovascular problems that make surgery risky.

Sex. Sex is probably not a major factor in determining prognosis. Studies which have examined whether sex is related to long-term outcome have had conflicting results.

Symptoms. Those patients who have no symptoms of colorectal cancer have a better five-year survival rate than those who do have symptoms. The duration of symptoms probably has little or no effect on prognosis. However, bleeding is one symptom that actually gives a better prognosis. It is hypothesized that this is so because tumors that bleed give an earlier "announcement" of their presence. The presence of bowel obstruction at the time of diagnosis reduces the chance that surgical cure can be obtained and reduces the five-year survival rate significantly. When the bowel has perforated (pierced through because of cancer), the outcome is very much worsened, and the likelihood of long-term survival is less than 10 percent. It is not certain that a longer duration of symptoms necessarily implies a worse stage and prognosis.

Stage. As stage of cancer increases, the long-term survival rate decreases. The status of the lymph nodes is perhaps the most important aspect of staging in relation to prognosis. This is because the lymph nodes are usually the first stage in transit of cancer cells to other sites, and the more lymph nodes involved at the time of surgery, the more forbidding the outcome. Involvement of adjacent organs makes for less favorable prognosis, but there are enough long-term survivors in this situation to warrant a surgeon still making a serious effort to remove the tumor in its entirety, even if that means removing adjacent organ tissue.

Vascular invasion. In a study by English pathologists of more than one thousand cases of colon cancer, 35 percent had cancerous involvement of nearby veins. If the veins were located within the bowel wall, the presence of cancer had no adverse effect on prognosis, but if the veins were located outside of the bowel wall, a poorer prognosis was observed.

Location of cancer. Rectal cancers generally have a poorer prognosis when compared to other locations of the colon. Conflicting opinions exist regarding whether right-sided colon cancers have a better prognosis than left-sided cancers.

Tumor size. Taken by itself, size of a colorectal cancer probably does not affect prognosis.

Tumor histology. Histology means microscopic anatomy. The more undifferentiated the cancer, the poorer the prognosis. If a cancer secretes large amounts of mucus, the prognosis may be less favorable. These types of cancers may be referred to as mucinous adenocarcinomas or as signet cell adenocarcinomas. Signet cell cancers are usually high grade and poorly differentiated. Cancers that have a hard feel due to formation of dense bands of scar tissue (known as scirrhous carcinoma) have a poorer prognosis.

Analysis of chromosome content. Extra chromosomes in cancer cells, a condition known as aneuploidy, as opposed to diploidy (normal chromosome number), is believed to be a predictor of more aggressive behavior and greater tendency to metastasize. Chromosome content (ploidy) analysis is a standard part of breast cancer evaluation, but is not used routinely for colon cancer prognostication. The value of ploidy analysis in standard treatment of colon cancer has not yet been fully established.

Analysis of genetic mutations. Damage to the DCC gene, located on chromosome 18, has been correlated with a negative impact on prognosis in patients with stage II or B colorectal cancer.

Prognosis by Stage

When all is said and done, the most important prognostic factor is the stage at the time of initial diagnosis. Other factors such as those listed above may influence prognosis by various degrees. Clinical judgment of the importance of these various factors must be exercised by the attending physicians, particularly if treatment decisions regarding surgery or adjuvant therapy need to be made.

In general, the higher the stage, the less favorable the prognosis. However, even if the stage is low, other indicators of aggressiveness may tilt the decision towards more aggressive therapy. Likewise, a higher-stage carcinoma with low aggressiveness may behave more favorably than a lower-stage cancer with more aggressive features. The following table of prognosis by stage is not absolute, and should be taken as only an approximation of real-life outcomes. It should always be remembered that these are statistical results. The individual response or result cannot be inferred absolutely from this table. The five-year survival rate is the most common yardstick used in oncology; this figure indicates the percentage of patients in a particular stage category who are still alive after five years of follow-up.

Table 6.3. Prognosis by Stage

Stage	5-Year Survival Rate
A	>90%
B$_I$	85%
B$_2$	70–75%
C	26–60 % (survival decreases with nodal involvement)
D	5%

How Colon Cancer Spreads (Metastasis)

Colon cancer becomes invasive when it penetrates the muscularis mucosa, where lymphatic vessels may be susceptible to infiltration by cancer cells. Growth of the cancer proceeds by further invasion deeper into the bowel wall and eventually into adjacent tissues. Thus, colorectal cancer grows more circumferentially (inward, deeper and radially) than longitudinally (superficially, outward into the lumen and lengthwise along the colon). If cancer grows rapidly and outstrips the growth of its own blood vessel supply, necrosis (death of tissue), ulceration, and bleeding may occur from the disrupted tissue.

Spread of cancer may then occur in five ways: via (1) lymphatics, (2) blood, (3) direct extension to other organs, (4) free intra-abdominal spread (drop metastases), and (5) spread within the lumen of the bowel (intraluminal spread). Cells that have broken free of the primary tumor mass invade lymphatics and veins, then spread to lymph nodes and other organs, especially the liver and the lung. The liver is the favored first site of metastasis, since blood in veins that drain the colon is subsequently drained by the liver before proceeding to the lung. Cancer can invade locally into adjacent (pericolonic or perirectal) fat or into local pelvic muscles or into nearby organs such as the prostate, bladder, vagina, uterus, ovaries, fallopian tube, small intestine, spleen, ureters, and pancreas. Cancer may directly spread along nerves, and this can result in pain.

Since the spread of cancer through the network of lymph nodes is believed to be an orderly and consecutive process, the appearance of cancer in adjacent lymph nodes does not preclude the possibility of cure. Simply stated, cancer may not yet have spread into the next group of nodes. Thus, a firm principle of colorectal cancer surgery is always to remove the adjacent regional lymph nodes of the affected part of the bowel. "Skip metastases," in which cancer cells are found in distant lymph nodes before they appear in nearby nodes, is unusual.

Spread of colorectal cancer cells via the bloodstream is possible once cancer has invaded the lamina propria, where there is an abundant supply of capillaries. Cancer cells may be found in the circulating blood with a remarkably high frequency, but the presence of cancer cells in the blood does not by itself predict metastasis. Blood is a notably inhospitable habitat for cancer cells. Cancer cells may survive in blood for only a short amount of time, and die before metastasizing to another organ. The occurrence of blood-borne metastasis requires that a number of nonrandom steps occur before cancer cells safely reach another organ, and many factors work against metastasis. One is that cancer cells vary in their propensity or ability to spread; another is that they must evade the natural immune system of the body; yet another is their need to somehow insinuate themselves into the deep tissues of another organ and develop a nurturing environment for themselves, through angiogenesis (development of blood vessels) and the elaboration of various growth factors, in unfamiliar territory. Thus, as in all biology, "fitness" determines which cancer cells survive and form metastatic colonies. Just as certain mutations favor the development of colorectal cancer, mutations also determine which cells metastasize.

Table 6.4. The Metastatic "Cascade"

Step-by-Step Analysis of How Cancer Spreads
(Adapted from DeVita, *Cancer: Principles and Practice of Oncology*, chapter 8)

Tumor initiation. Carcinogenesis begins; mutations lead to oncogene activation or tumor suppressor gene inactivation (or both).

Promotion, progression, and proliferation. Further genetic instability. Growth factors permit tumor proliferation. Disabling of the apoptosis process.

Angiogenesis. Development of new blood supply for the growing cancer; this is aided by various growth factors (hormones or proteins which stimulate growth of tumor-supplying blood vessels).

Invasion of local tissues, blood, and lymph vessels.

Spread out of blood into other tissue. Requires "stickiness" of cancer cells in the blood to tissues outside of the bloodstream. These cells then "unstick" themselves and migrate through the foreign tissue to form "colonies" within the deeper layers of tissue. Further angiogenesis needed for growth of metastatic colonies.

Evasion of "host" defenses. Cancer cells must have a way to fight the cells of the immune system; mutations may occur which permit the overcoming of these natural defense systems and may also permit resistance to treatment with chemotherapy (known as drug-resistance genes).

Once colon cancer has penetrated through the outer surface of the bowel wall, cancer cells may by free implantation ("drop metastases") spread within the abdomen and grow. Drop metastases, though not very common, may develop from tumor cells that have shed from the primary tumor site into the open cavity of the abdomen, and may implant on any surface within the abdomen. Cells that land and grow on the surface of the lining tissue of the abdomen, the peritoneum, may cause the development of fluid accumulation within the abdomen known as ascites.

The fifth route is spread of cancer cells by free implantation within the lumen to other sites of bowel mucosa. The spillage of cancer cells within the lumen at the time of surgery may account for postoperative recurrence of cancer at the site of anastomosis (where the ends of bowel are reconnected after surgery). This is referred to as anastomotic recurrence.

7. Surgical Treatment of Colon Cancer

As with nearly every other form of cancer, cure of colorectal cancer begins with surgery. The surgeon will do the following:

1. Obtain preoperative blood tests (especially "tumor markers" such as CEA) to provide a baseline, or benchmark, for cancer staging (see chapter 5).
2. Make a careful assessment of the patient's medical ability to undergo surgery.
3. Remove the entire cancer, along with the vascular supply, lymphatics, and mesentery associated with that portion of the colon, with adequate "margins." (The margin is the amount of normal tissue left between the border of the cancerous tissue and the edge of the tissue removed.)
4. Remove adequate surrounding tissues (such as fat, lymph nodes, or adjacent organ tissue which may have the appearance of being involved) to establish whether there is any cancerous invasion.
5. Carefully examine other parts of the colon and rectum for coexisting cancers. The use of intraoperative colonoscopy or assistance of laparoscopy may be required.
6. Carefully inspect neighboring tissues and other abdominal organs (especially the liver) for evidence of cancer. If suspicious areas are detected, they must be biopsied by the surgeon for definitive determination of whether cancer has spread or not.

7. Minimize the long-term medical and psychological consequences of surgery without compromising the basic goal of attempting surgical cure.
8. Provide the pathologist with adequate material to determine the depth of invasion of the cancer and the extent of spread to lymph nodes and surrounding tissues.

The Incision

The location of the incision made by the surgeon is determined by several factors, not the least of which is the habit and preference of the person who performs the operation. However, location of the abdominal incision is influenced considerably by the location of the cancer itself.

Most often, an incision is made vertically in the middle of the abdomen (a midline incision). This permits a fair amount of flexibility for extension of the incision if required. Horizontal (transverse) incisions are occasionally made. These may be used in the case of a right colon cancer (right transverse incision, parallel to the lower border of the right rib cage) or a cancer of the splenic flexure (left subcostal transverse incision). In the case of a cancer that is low in the pelvis area, the midline incision may have to be extended down into the pelvis area.

Once the abdomen is opened, the surgeon performs a careful exploration and palpation (examination by touch) of the structures within the abdomen. In particular, the liver must be looked at and palpated with care, and, in women, the pelvic organs must be inspected.

During surgery, colonoscopy may be employed so that the physician can examine the internal portion of the colon to verify the location of a polyp or cancer. This may be helpful in planning the removal of the appropriate part of the bowel.

Types of Colon Cancer Operations

A number of "standard" resections are used by surgeons in the the treatment of colon cancer. These standard operations are based upon anatomic considerations, particularly the blood supply and lymphatic drainage of the different portions of the large bowel. (The circulation to the colon is described in chapter 2.)

En bloc resection is the term applied to an operation in which the affected bowel, blood, lymph supply, mesentery, and any affected adjacent tissues are all removed. The major artery supplying an affected portion of bowel is usually ligated (tied off with a suture) at its origin from the aorta. Traditionally, the margin length has been five centimeters (two inches).

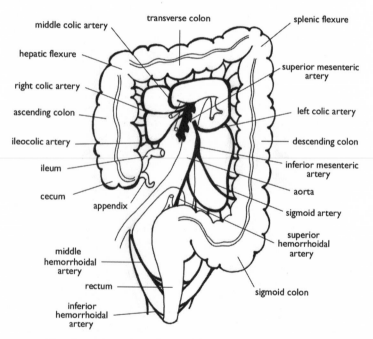

FIG. 7.I. Blood supply to the colon and rectum.

Table 7.1. Types of Surgical Procedures for Colon Cancer

Operation	Area of Colon Treated	Technique	Comments
Right hemicolectomy	Right, or ascending, colon	Right colic and ileocolic blood vessels, as well as the hepatic branch of the middle colic artery, are ligated.	
Transverse colon resection	Transverse colon	Depends on whether the right, middle, or left portion is involved. Middle colic and either right colic or left colic arteries are ligated.	Sometimes necessitates removal of right colon. Stomach, duodenum, pancreas, and spleen are at risk of injury. Greater omentum is included in the resection.

continued

Table 7.1. (Continued)

Operation	Area of Colon Treated	Technique	Comments
Left hemicolectomy	Splenic flexure and descending colon	Splenic branch of middle colic artery and left colic artery are ligated.	Anastomosis (reconnection) is made between transverse colon and sigmoid colon. Ureter, gonadal blood vessels, spleen, and pancreas are at risk of injury.
Sigmoid colectomy	Sigmoid colon	Sigmoidal and left colic arteries are ligated.	
Anterior resection of rectosigmoid	Distal (far-end) sigmoid and proximal (near-end) rectal cancers	Peritoneum freed, rectum is detached from sacrum (tailbone).	Ureters, gonadal and iliac blood vessels, and nerves to bladder and genitals are at risk of injury.

| Proctectomy | Cancers low in the rectum, two to three centimeters from the anus | | |
| Abdomino-perineal resection (AP resection, or Miles procedure) | Rectal cancers which are attached to the *sphincter* (ring of muscle tissue that permits opening and closure of the anus) | Performed in two phases: abdominal and perineal. May require two teams of surgeons. Abdominal phase proceeds like low anterior resection. | Requires formation of permanent colostomy, since the sphincter cannot be preserved. Anus sewn shut during perineal phase of surgery. |

Possible Complications of Surgery

The potential complications of surgery are many and potentially dismaying. If one forgets that all medical interventions are inherently risky (but never performed when the potential risk outweighs the potential benefit), the option to refuse surgical intervention may seem attractive. The same kind of rational thinking needs to be applied when patients and physicians discuss adjunctive therapies for colorectal cancer, such as radiation and chemotherapy.

The complications of surgery include blood loss and subsequent requirement for blood transfusion. This is rare in operations in the upper abdomen, but those performed in the lower abdominal/pelvic (AP) area can easily be complicated by hemorrhage, even in the hands of the most painstaking and experienced surgeon.

Infection both of the wound and the abdominal cavity can occur, again, even when scrupulous technique is performed. Situations that may predispose to infection include an impaired immune system and incomplete cleansing of the bowel before surgery. The development of newer and more potent antibiotics and their use before and during surgery have helped reduce infection rates considerably. A complication referred to as wound dehiscence involves the surgical wound failing to heal properly and coming apart.

Leakage from the anastomosis (the rejoined ends of bowel after the cancer-containing portion has been removed), also known as anastomotic leak, can result in postoperative pain and infection. This complication is more common in low anterior resections, and may require the temporary creation of a colostomy. The increasing use of stapling devices in bowel surgery has led to a higher rate of stenosis (narrowing) and potential blockage. This situation may require dilation or surgical revision of the anastomosis.

Damage to the ureters (the tubular structures that connect the kidneys to the bladder) can occur during colorectal surgery. This could potentially lead to blockage and infection of the kidneys and the urinary tract.

Bowel obstruction can result from adhesions (tough bands of scar tissue that may develop after abdominal surgery and cause abnormal joining of normally separate loops of bowel) or from tension and torsion on the bowel created by reconnection (anastomosis).

AP resection can result in impotence, retrograde ejaculation (semen is discharged backward into the bladder) in men, urinary dysfunction, serious wound infection, and even death.

Possible Complications from Colostomy

The skin surrounding the stoma (opening) may become irritated and chafed (excoriated). Actual infection, with skin bacteria such as *Staphylococcus* and *Streptococcus* or with yeast, can complicate this type of excoriation. Infections internal to the stoma, and even abscess inside of the abdomen, can occur. Weakening of the abdominal wall muscles may result in outpouching of the abdomen around the stoma (hernia). The stoma itself may herniate and push outward (prolapse). Strictures of the stoma and obstruction of the small bowel may occur. Fistulas (abnormal passages) between the internal part of the colostomy and the external abdomen or even between the internal colostomy and adjacent small bowel can also occur.

Special Surgical Considerations

Preparation for Radiation Therapy

Radiation therapy is often used as an adjunct to surgery in cancers of the rectum. In order to reduce or prevent unwanted complications from radiation, the surgeon may move loops of the small bowel out of the way of the radiation field. The surgeon may also leave surgical clips that are visible on x-ray so that the radiation therapist may more accurately map out the field to which radiation will be given.

Local Excision of Rectal Cancer and Sphincter-Saving Operations

The desire to preserve the anal sphincter, and thereby permit the patient to retain control of defecation, has been of concern to surgical oncologists. In recent years, the belief that surgical control of some cancers in the rectum could not be accomplished without sacrificing the sphincter has been challenged by the performing of operations that preserve the sphincter function. In addition, the desire to avoid some of the more serious side effects of the AP resection has led to an interest in finding other ways to perform adequate surgery.

Transanal removal of cancers has been found to be a successful procedure when used with strict selection criteria. This operation has the serious limitation of not permitting visualization of the lymph nodes and lymphatic vessel status, but it does offer the advantage of permitting a potentially curative procedure for persons who are too medically fragile for an AP resection. Criteria for this procedure include: (1) the cancer is small, not rigidly fixed to tissue; (2) the cancer is less than ten centimeters from the anal verge; (3) the cancer is located away from the vagina; (4) the cancer does not have an aggressive appearance on the biopsy; (5) there is no evidence of lymph node metastases; and (6) the cancer has a nonulcerated appearance. Endoluminal rectal ultrasound is useful for determining depth of the cancer and whether there is involvement of lymph nodes.

Techniques used for the removal of these cancers include traditional surgical excision, laser destruction, cautery, or radiation. Transrectal endoluminal microsurgery is available in a few specialized centers, and permits precise excision of rectal cancers.

Multimodality therapy utilizing the above techniques, plus radiation therapy and chemotherapy, may permit less debilitating operations to be performed even in high-risk situations for rectal cancer. This would include situations in which microscopic cancer metastases are already likely at the time of diagnosis.

Total Mesenteric Excision (TME) for Rectal Cancer

TME is a surgical technique introduced in the 1980s for treatment of rectal cancer. Surgical techniques are employed which require sharper dissection (or removal of tissue) than conventional surgical approaches. Use of this method results in complete removal of the rectum with its closely surrounding tissue intact. Some surgical authorities have reported that this technique produces lower rates of impotence, bladder dysfunction, and recurrence of cancer than conventional surgical techniques that use "blunt" techniques of dissection.

Removal of the Ovaries (Oophorectomy)

There is a small chance that colon cancer may involve the ovaries. The probability is higher in premenopausal women. If one ovary is involved, there is a greater than 50 percent likelihood that the other ovary is also. Involvement may be by direct physical contact and invasion, or by spread of cancer cells to the ovaries through the bloodstream. Therefore, the possibility that the ovaries may need to be removed must be discussed before surgery.

Some authorities suggest that prophylactic (preventive) removal of the ovaries should be considered routinely in all premenopausal women with colon cancer.

Bowel Obstruction

The occurrence of bowel obstruction may be as high as 25 percent. It is more commonly seen in the elderly and in women.

Left-sided obstructive colorectal carcinoma can be managed surgically by a multistaged approach or a single-stage
approach. The Hartmann procedure is a two-stage approach
that is preferred by some surgeons. In the first stage, the
cancer is resected and the proximal colon is turned into a
colostomy. The distal colon is sutured or stapled off. In the
second stage, the two ends are reconnected to reestablish
bowel continuity. Single-stage approaches to obstructing left
colon cancer in the descending colon or proximal sigmoid
colon include: (1) subtotal colectomy with ileorectal anastomosis (connect the small bowel to the rectum) or ileosigmoid
anastomosis (connect the small bowel to the sigmoid colon),
and (2) "on the table" bowel preparation with resection and
reanastomosis. In the latter procedure, the appendix is removed and a flexible tube (catheter) is inserted into the bowel
that is then irrigated with saline solution ("mechanical prep")
before removal of the affected portion of bowel.

If obstruction is found in the ascending (right) or transverse colon, a single-stage procedure can be performed.

Perforation of the Bowel

This surgical emergency can result in peritonitis or localized abscess. Perforation (puncturing open) of the bowel
can occur proximal to an obstructing carcinoma or may be
caused by direct invasion of the cancer. Immediate surgery
is required and careful lavage (irrigation or washing out)
of the abdominal cavity, along with drainage of any pus or
abscess material and administration of antibiotics, is necessary.
In spite of these measures, the morbidity (debilitation and
prolonged convalescence) and mortality which ensue under
this situation can be high.

Neighboring Organ Involvement

In about 10 percent of cases, direct extension of cancer to a
bordering organ may be seen. In spite of that, cure rates may

still be high when surgery is extended to include the involved adjacent tissue. In some cases, a fistula (hollow passage) may connect the colon to the neighboring tissue, or the connection may be via scar tissue known as adhesions.

The Role of Surgery in Metastatic Disease

In some situations even where cancer has spread to the liver or the lung, surgery may still be helpful.

Liver metastases. When there is one or only a few metastases to the liver, and there is no sign of cancer elsewhere, it is reasonable to remove them. This is particularly so if the blood CEA is not elevated and if there has been a long interval since the original surgery. A surgeon may observe a patient for some months before performing liver resection; this is to be more certain that small nodules of cancer beneath the level of detection do not exist and appear later. Prognosis may be greatly improved when such an approach is taken.

Lung metastases. The likelihood of metastases to the lung is greater with cancers of the rectum than with other colon cancers. This is because some of the veins that drain the rectum lead directly to the lungs. Like liver metastases, the possibility of performing resection of such metastases is good when there is only a solitary lesion at the time the primary lesion in the colon or rectum is discovered, or when there has been a long interval from the initial surgery.

Palliative resection. Even when colorectal cancer has spread outside of the colon and is felt to be incurable, removal of the primary cancer may still be justified. This would be the case if the primary site of cancer was causing (or could potentially cause) obstruction, hemorrhage, or pain. A judgment may have to be made as to whether a person will survive long enough to have such complications, and whether an operation is fitting or not, particularly if it would result in colostomy.

Laparoscopic Procedures

The development of laparoscopy for different types of surgery (gallbladder, hernia, and gynecologic operations, to name a few) has introduced a new age of surgery. Laparoscopic surgery may permit smaller incisions, shorter hospitalization, less disfigurement, and quicker return to normal activity. Laparoscopy makes use of a tiny video camera that is inserted through a small incision into the abdomen and permits surgical procedures to be performed while action is monitored on video cameras in the operating room. Carbon dioxide is used to inflate the abdominal cavity. This permits the surgeon to explore the contents inside the abdomen and safely perform electric cautery.

Laparoscopy is available also for colon resections, but indications for using it are limited. Laparoscopy may be used for performing the entire procedure, or it may be used as a technical assistance for an open procedure. Preliminary reports indicate that laparoscopic techniques for performing colon cancer resection compare favorably to traditional open procedures, but further clinical trials are warranted before this type of surgery is accepted as being equal to traditional open procedures.

Types of colon operations that may be performed by laparoscopy include hemicolectomy, anterior and low anterior resections, and creation of colostomies and ileostomies. Other colon operations that may be performed with the assistance of laparoscopy include abdomino-perineal resections and primary anastomosis procedures.

Those patients who may be too fragile for standard laparotomy may be eligible for laparoscopy, as are patients in whom standard endoscopic polypectomy cannot be performed because of the possibility of fragmentation of the tissue during the procedure. Patients with small tumors in the right side of the colon may be candidates for laparoscopic procedures.

Sometimes when a segment of the bowel can be resected more easily than having a biopsy performed by endoscopy, laparoscopy may be the appropriate procedure. This applies when it is not known whether the bowel harbors benign or malignant tissue. If cancer is found, a decision may have to be made as to whether the operation should be converted to a traditional, open laparotomy (surgical opening of the abdomen).

We do not yet know whether laparoscopic surgery yields the same long-term results as conventional laparotomy for colon cancer. Concerns have been raised that during laparoscopic colorectal cancer surgery cancer cells may be implanted where the incision is made or may be disbursed during the procedure. Certainly, the conservative decision would be to take a conventional open surgical approach. However, special circumstances (which above all include the experience and training of the surgeon and any unique conditions that may affect the patient's ability to undergo conventional laparotomy) should always be taken into consideration at the time of surgery before a final decision is made.

Citing a number of concerns, including those mentioned above, the National Institute of Clinical Evidence (United Kingdom) issued a statement in December 2000 recommending against the use of laparoscopic (or "keyhole") surgery for colorectal cancer.

8. Treatment of Later Stages of Colon Cancer

Adjuvant Therapy

The mainstay of treatment for colon cancer has been surgery. If the cancer has not spread into lymph nodes, does not show other unfavorable characteristics (such as full penetration of the bowel wall or perforation of the bowel), and has not spread to other organs, surgery is usually all that is needed.

Observations of thousands of cases of colorectal cancer over many decades have proven that as the stage of colon cancer increases, the likelihood of recurrence increases and the prospect for cure diminishes. This has led to extensive investigation of the usefulness of adjuvant therapies. "Adjuvant" simply means that which assists or improves another treatment.

Cancer metastasizes when cells from the primary cancer site travel via blood or lymphatic vessels or direct invasion to other sites in the body. Before surgery has been performed to remove the primary mass of cancer, some cells must have "escaped" to fertile ground elsewhere in the body. Therefore, the theory behind adjuvant therapy is that if some form of additional treatment can kill off the remaining few cancer cells, then the chance of cancer spread or recurrence can be diminished. The term used for these undetectable cancer cells is microscopic metastases.

The Holy Grail for almost thirty years of colorectal cancer research was an adjuvant therapy that would be effective in improving survival rates. This search was largely pursued through chemotherapy drugs, especially 5-FU, with the hope that a drug or a combination of drugs would provide the key.

In the late 1980s this grail was finally found when researchers reported preliminary results of a study which showed that a combination of 5-FU, a drug first developed and used in the 1950s, and levamisole (a drug used to kill worms in animals) was effective in reducing the rate of relapse of stage C_2 colon cancer and improving the survival rates. 5-FU is called a fluoropyrimidine because of the fluorine atom that has been synthetically attached to the uracil molecule, a component of RNA. 5-FU was the first "designer drug" used for cancer chemotherapy and was synthesized by Dr. Charles Heidelberger at the University of Wisconsin in the early 1950s. He made use of the observation that cancer cells in rats use uracil more avidly than normal cells and postulated that this difference could be exploited to a therapeutic advantage. 5-FU differs from uracil by having a flourine atom where a hydrogen atom should normally be present. 5-FU may then exert its antitumor effect through several mechanisms affecting both DNA and RNA.

The exact mechanism by which levamisole works is not known, but it is believed that the drug acts as a "modulator" (or activator) of the human immune system to fight cancer cells. By itself, it appears not to have significant cancer-fighting activity. However, it is effective when combined with 5-FU.

In 1995 final results of the study were published, and these showed that the survival rate of stage III or C_2 colon cancer patients who were treated with 5-FU and levamisole after surgery was 60 percent, versus 46 percent for those who did not receive the treatment. The major side effects of this treatment include mild liver dysfunction, neurotoxicity (memory disturbances, wobbly gait, confusion, and depression), taste alteration, and achy joints. The combination of 5-FU and levamisole (which had been quickly accepted as a standard treatment by the early 1990s) was later superseded by another combination, 5-FU and leucovorin, in the early-to-mid 1990s. Leucovorin is a chemical relative of folic acid, an essential nutrient, or vitamin. Leucovorin is also felt to be a modulator, which augments the action of other drugs such as 5-FU. The combination of 5-FU and leucovorin was originally used for patients with widespread metastases, and then it was found active as an adjuvant therapy (see below).

The benefit of adjuvant chemotherapy for patients with Dukes B_2 colon cancers has never been fully substantiated by a clinical trial. Some studies have indeed shown a small survival advantage, but when scrutinized carefully by statisticians this small advantage appears to be a random outcome. Nevertheless, some, if not many, medical oncologists use some form of adjuvant chemotherapy for these lesions.

Although treatment with 5-FU and leucovorin is generally well tolerated by most patients, many side effects may occur. Cells of the body which are growing more rapidly than others

Table 8.1. Adjuvant Chemotherapy Protocols for C_2 Colon Cancer

5FU plus Leucovorin (A)

5-FU 425 mg/m² intravenous push daily for 5 days	Repeat every 4–5 weeks for 6 cycles
Leucovorin 20 mg/m² intravenous push daily for 5 days	

5-FU plus Leucovorin (B)

Leucovorin 500 mg/m² intravenous infusion over 2 hours followed by	Weekly for 6 weeks followed by 3 weeks rest. Repeat 4–6 cycles.
5-FU 500 mg/m² intravenous bolus	

(such as hair, skin, mucous tissue cells, and bone marrow) and therefore probably have active DNA production are more likely to be affected by chemotherapy drugs than other tissues. This is why, like many other chemotherapy drugs, 5-FU causes depression of bone marrow activity leading to (1) anemia, (2) lowering of the white blood cell count (neutropenia), which can result in diminished immune function, and (3) low platelet count (thrombocytopenia), which can lead to bleeding and easy bruising. Blood counts are monitored closely during chemotherapy to ensure that counts are not dangerously low. Anemia can be treated with a red-cell-growth-stimulating hormone known as erythropoietin (Procrit). Neutropenia can be treated with white-blood-cell-stimulating factors known as G-CSF (Neupogen) or GM-CSF (Leukine). Thrombocytopenia can be observed if it is not severe, or treated with a growth factor oprelvekin (Neumega), or treated with a transfusion of platelets. Diarrhea is a frequent but generally tolerable effect of 5-FU. It can usually be managed with over-the-counter medications such as Kaopectate (parapectolin) and Immodium (loperamide) or with prescription drugs such as Lomotil (diphenoxylate). To reduce toxicity caused by diarrhea, it is important that a patient consume large quantities of fluids to avoid dehydration.

Mucositis (irritation of mucous lining tissues in the mouth and throat) can be one of the most bothersome side effects of 5-FU. Treatment with mouthwashes and oral antibiotic solutions may be required. If diarrhea and mucositis are very severe, hospitalization may even be necessary to treat the dehydration and malnutrition that may ensue. Irritation of tear ducts (lacrimitis), causing redness and easy tearing or running of the eyes, may require treatment with antihistamine eye drops or tablets. Hair loss (alopecia) from 5-FU is mild or moderate. Complete hair loss from 5-FU alone is distinctly unusual. Nausea and vomiting (emesis) is in general a mild to moderate side effect. It is usually easily controlled or prevented with antiemetic medications such as Compazine (prochlorperazine), Decadron (dexamethasone), Zofran (ondansetron), Kytril (granisetron), and Anzemet (dolasetron). Nausea, vomiting, diarrhea, bone marrow depression, and mucositis may be particularly severe in a minority of patients who have a deficiency of an enzyme, DPD, which metabolizes and breaks down the 5-FU molecule (see below). Leucovorin is relatively safe and side effect free, severe allergy being the only major toxicity in a slim minority of patients.

Adjuvant therapy for rectal cancer involves the use of radiation. It is often combined with the drug 5-FU, which acts as a radiation sensitizer. That is, the 5-FU causes the cancer cells to become more sensitive to radiation. The basic mechanism of 5-FU radiation sensitization is not well understood. It is believed that 5-FU and similar drugs cause production of free radicals within DNA which are very damaging to the cell when exposed to radiation.

Other forms of adjuvant therapy for colon cancer have been tried. It is theorized that portal vein infusion, in which chemotherapy drugs are infused into the vein that feeds into the liver, helps kill or retard the growth of liver metastases. Benefit from this form of treatment has not been proven, and at this time it remains an investigational therapy. Immunotherapy with various agents such as the drug interferon, monoclonal antibodies to colon cancer cells, and vaccines have been or are being investigated (see chapter 10).

Interferons are proteins produced by many types of cells when they are exposed to a virus or other foreign DNA. They cause uninfected cells to produce a protein that interferes with the replication of foreign DNA. Interferons were developed as commercial drugs in the 1980s when a new type of biotechnology (known as recombinant DNA technology) was developed which allowed mass production of human interferons. Interferons have been found to fight certain types of cancer as well as certain viral infections. Unfortunately the addition of interferon to standard chemotherapy regimens has no apparent benefit in colorectal cancer and significantly increases side effects.

Deciding Who Gets Adjuvant Therapy

All patients with Dukes C_2 (or stage III) colon cancer should strongly consider having adjuvant chemotherapy. Since the 5-FU and leucovorin regimen is given for only six months, there is very little reason to give the 5-FU and levamisole regimen, which requires one year of administration.

It should be remembered that no study has shown a definite benefit from adjuvant treatment for patients with B_2 lesions (stage II). As mentioned above, it is likely that clinical practice in many communities and centers throughout the United States includes the recommendation for adjuvant chemotherapy for B_2 lesions. A patient who has this stage of colon cancer should carefully weigh the options, including risks and benefits of treatment, with the oncologist. Difficult treatment decisions such as this can sometimes be decided with the help of tumor boards, meetings of cancer specialists from different fields (pathology, surgery, radiation therapy, and medical oncology) which are held regularly at hospitals and medical centers that provide cancer treatment.

In the future, molecular and genetic factors (including specific chromosomal alterations) may identify patients at high risk of colon cancer relapse. This may afford greater selectivity in decisions regarding who would derive benefit from adjuvant chemotherapy (see chapter 10).

Therapy for Advanced Stage Disease

In advanced stage disease, cancer has spread to other organs outside of the colon. In particular, the liver and lung are frequent sites of cancer spread. Other possible sites of cancer spread include the peritoneum and organs adjacent to the bowel. Other distant sites of blood-borne metastasis, usually occurring late in the disease process, are bone and brain. (Theories of metastasis and spread of colon cancer are discussed in chapter 6.) If metastases are solitary or very few, surgical removal of them may be possible and may provide long-term remission. If metastases are many or diffuse (meaning that they cannot be picked out surgically because too many parts of an organ or several organs are involved) then the only reasonable option is chemotherapy.

5-FU

The mainstay of chemotherapy for advanced colorectal cancer is 5-FU, which is taken up by cells and can incorporate into either RNA or DNA. It may be broken down by an enzyme known as dihydropyrimidine dehydrogenase (DPD); about 6 percent of people have a deficiency of this enzyme, which can result in much greater toxicity of the drug, including severe diarrhea, mouth sores, bone marrow depression, and nerve toxicity, since more of the drug is available for incorporation into DNA and RNA. On the other hand, elevated levels of DPD in cancer cells may reduce the effectiveness of the drug. Action of 5-FU is also partly dependent upon another enzyme known as thymidilate synthase. 5-FU is converted to the metabolite FdUMP (fluoro-deoxyuridine monophosphate) which binds to thymidine monophosphate, a molecule essential for DNA synthesis. Tumors that do not show much activity of this enzyme may have little or no response to the effect of 5-FU.

5-FU has been used in a number of ways, each one designed to take advantage of an aspect of the drug's pharmacology that could possibly give a therapeutic advantage. It is not well absorbed by the gut, so it is nearly always administered intravenously, but it may be infused in different ways. It may be given rapidly (as bolus), or over a period of

twenty-four or more hours, in which presumably the tumor
is exposed to the drug for a longer time. When given as a
bolus, it may be preferentially incorporated into RNA, while
protracted infusions may act upon DNA through thymidilate
synthase. For many years 5-FU given alone was the only
chemotherapy that showed any benefit to patients with advanced colorectal cancer. The odds of 5-FU alone causing
a response or improvement in survival are only about 15
percent, however.

5-FU Combinations

5-FU has been combined with other drugs in an effort to
improve its efficacy. The combination of 5-FU and levamisole
for adjuvant therapy is described above. Levamisole enhances
immune system activity, but the mechanism by which it works
together with 5-FU to achieve greater affects is not known.

Leucovorin acts by helping stabilize complexes of thymidilate synthase and FdUMP. This results in increased toxicity
of 5-FU to the cancer cell. 5-FU and leucovorin has been
the standard treatment regimen for many years for patients
with metastatic colorectal cancer. It is easy to administer
as an outpatient treatment, and is relatively nontoxic. The
percentage of patients who show reduction in tumor size with
this combination is about thirty to thirty-five.

Irinotecan (Camptosar)

Irinotecan is a partially synthetic drug that originates from
plant material. It works by inhibiting an enzyme called topoisomerase I, which helps to stabilize the double helix structure
of DNA. Because of the higher rate of DNA production in
tumors, the concentration of this enzyme in cancer cells is
about fifteen times that of normal cells. Therefore, cancer
cells are more sensitive to its action than normal cells. Irinotecan causes the helical strands of DNA to destabilize and
break apart, causing cell death. This drug has been found to

be very effective in treating patients with advanced colorectal cancer, even those who have failed previous treatment with 5-FU. In one study, the survival rate in patients receiving irinotecan after failing initial 5-FU treatment was 13 percent higher than in those who received another treatment with 5-FU (45 percent versus 32 percent).

Irinotecan has also been combined with 5-FU and leucovorin and compared to the combination of 5-FU and leucovorin alone. The three-drug regimen showed better results than the two-drug course. In the future we may see this three-drug regimen replace 5-FU/leucovorin as the first line of treatment for advanced colorectal cancer. Like other chemotherapy, irinotecan may be given as an outpatient treatment, and is administered on either a weekly or a twenty-one-day schedule. It can cause significant diarrhea, and may require use of the antidote drug atropine to control this problem. In some cases, irinotecan may cause metabolic derangement serious enough to require a patient's hospitalization.

New Forms of 5-FU

The development of newer forms of 5-FU in recent years is changing the way in which metastatic colorectal cancer will be treated and how adjuvant chemotherapy is given. One adaptation is the creation of 5-FU molecules that can inhibit DPD; an example of a drug that is modified in such a manner is eniluracil.

Capecitabine (Xeloda) is a commercially available "new" form of 5-FU, also known as a 5-FU "prodrug" because it does not become the active drug until it is acted upon in the body. It ultimately ends up as 5-FU in cells. In contrast to 5-FU, it can be given orally. It was designed to be absorbed through the gastrointestinal tract unchanged and then to undergo conversion in the liver into cancer-fighting form. In bypassing metabolism in the gastrointestinal tract, the gastrointestinal toxicity of 5-FU is reduced considerably.

Capecitabine is converted in the liver to a molecule called 5-deoxy-5-fluoridine (5-DFUR), which is then taken up by tumor cells and converted to 5-FU, where its concentration is extremely high compared to normal tissues. 5-FU is then converted to its active metabolite FdUMP. The stability of capecitabine as a therapeutic drug lies in the fact that the enzymes which convert it to 5-FU are highly active in cancer cells. The toxicity of treatment is therefore much less compared to that of 5-FU itself. The most significant toxicity of capecitabine involves peeling and redness of the skin of the hands and feet, referred to as hand-foot syndrome.

Ftorafur is another 5-FU prodrug that can be given orally. It is converted in the liver to 5-FU. Its use is limited because it is active only for a short time and because it can damage nerves.

UFT is a combination of uracil and ftorafur. Uracil is also broken down by DPD; therefore, the addition of uracil to the compound slows the breakdown of ftorafur by DPD and prolongs its activity. Side effects include diarrhea, abdominal cramps, nausea, and vomiting.

Other New Drugs

Oxaliplatin is approved and in use in Europe, but has been rejected by the U.S. Food and Drug Administration because studies have not yet shown it to have a survival advantage. This drug is related to other platinum-complex drugs already in use, cisplatin and carboplatin, but has less toxicity. These drugs work by binding to DNA in ways that decrease its synthesis.

Raltitrexed (Tomudex) is a folic acid derivative that inhibits the enzyme thymidilate synthase.

Trimetrexate (Neutrexin) interferes with DNA synthesis by antagonizing the action of folic acid; it was originally designed for use against malaria and has also been effective for treatment of *Pnemocystis carinii* pneumonia, a type of opportunistic infection found frequently in patients with

AIDS. In some studies, it has been shown to enhance the effectiveness of the 5-FU/leucovorin combination; it may also have effectiveness as a single drug treatment.

Hepatic Arterial Infusion

This technique uses a form of 5-FU known as FudR (fluorodeoxyuridine) that is directly infused into the liver via the hepatic artery to treat metastases. The liver receives blood from both the hepatic artery and the portal vein, but cancer cells in the liver appear to receive blood preferentially from the hepatic artery. While this treatment may afford an opportunity to shrink lesions in the liver, it has not gained wide acceptance because of the technical difficulties of the procedure and the cost of the pump that provides drug delivery. In addition, it is not clear that this treatment produces a survival advantage. However, a recent study from the Memorial Sloan-Kettering Cancer Center in New York *did* show improved survival rates in a group of patients who received this type of therapy in combination with conventional intravenous chemotherapy (after having surgical resection of liver metastases) compared with a similar group of patients who only received conventional chemotherapy.

Adjuvant Therapy for Rectal Cancer

Treatment of rectal cancer requires an approach that is different from those used in other colon cancers. Rectal cancer is more likely to recur locally and in adjacent tissues because it is more difficult for surgeons to obtain wide surgical margins in the relatively small space of the pelvis. Radiation therapy therefore reduces recurrence of rectal cancer locally, and, if given preoperatively (neoadjuvant therapy), may reduce the need for a sphincter-destroying operation. Chemotherapy given as neoadjuvant therapy along with radiation may improve response and treatment effect.

9. Prevention

The concept of colon cancer prevention (and perhaps elimination) is not a radical one, nor is it unrealistic. Furthermore, prevention of colorectal cancer could have momentous public health and economic impact on the United States, where as many as 140,000 people each year are diagnosed with this disease.

The conjecture that colon cancer is preventable is based on several notable and unique features of this disease. Colon cancer originates from the mucosal layer of the bowel, which is completely accessible to visual inspection by means of endoscopy. The forerunner of colon cancer is the polyp in as many as 85 percent of cases. This can be both discovered and liquidated at one sitting. People who have polyps can be kept under surveillance for development of future polyps. In addition, there is a long period of time between the first stages of colon cancer development and the stage at which it becomes symptomatic, providing the opportunity to screen for and remove the diseased cells before they spread.

Moreover, epidemiological studies strongly suggest that diet is a factor in the pathogenesis of colon cancer, as described in chapter 1. If this is true, then dietary change on a population-wide scale should reduce the incidence of colon cancer, and individual attention to diet should provide personal benefit as well.

The progression of benign changes in the bowel mucosa to malignancy is well understood. The genetic changes that propel the step-by-step development of cancer are also being mapped out. Thus, prevention may be aimed at one or more of the steps leading to cancer. Testing for genetic markers of this disease is available, albeit in crude form, and in the future may help patients and doctors predict colon cancer development.

Finally, a number of studies are showing that aspirin and other medications that inhibit the synthesis of prostaglandins (known as nonsteroidal anti-inflammatory drugs, or NSAIDs, and COX inhibitors) may prevent the development of polyps. Certain other substances such as the vitamin folic acid may reduce the incidence of colon cancer by other means.

Diet

Diet seems to influence colorectal carcinogenesis in two ways. On the one hand, dietary fat is presumed to have a cancer-promoting effect. On the other, dietary fiber is thought to have a protective effect.

The ingestion of fat in the diet stimulates release of bile. Bile is secreted from the liver and enters the gallbladder where it becomes much more concentrated. In response to meals containing fat, the gallbladder releases bile into the small intestine. Bile serves to dissolve cholesterol and the breakdown products of fat digestion in the small bowel and help the absorption of these substances into the blood. Bile is thought to be a factor in the development of colon cancer. People who have had the gallbladder removed may have a higher incidence of colon cancer.

Medical researchers theorize that fatty acids and bile cause irritation of the bowel mucosa, which in turn leads to increased proliferation of cells with abnormal DNA (genetic mutations) and eventual cancer. Cell damage may be promoted by the generation of free radicals caused by peroxidation of fat. Free radicals are atoms with unpaired electrons or protons. They are highly reactive and can cause damage when they combine with cellular components. In another theory, it is postulated that excessive concentrations of a substance known as diacylglycerol, which causes overgrowth and eventual malignancy of cells, may result from interactions of fatty acids, bile, and intestinal bacteria.

Africans are known to have a low rate of colon cancer, which is likely due to their diet being high in fiber and unrefined food. A study that compared the incidence of colon cancer in New York City inhabitants with that of people in Finland found that Finns have a lower rate of the disease, although they consume similar amounts of fat per capita. The difference seems to be that the Finnish people consume much more fiber than do New Yorkers. Thus, people in the Big Apple would fare better if they ate more big apples.

What is fiber? It is a group of complex plant substances such as cellulose that are resistant to breakdown by human digestive enzymes. Pectin and gums, which are soluble, are included in the definition because they have fiber-like effects on the digestive tract. In fact, a number of bulk laxatives are composed largely of gums.

Other studies of both humans and animals have supported the theory that increased dietary fiber reduces colon cancer development. Fiber is believed to bind bile and keep it from coming into contact with the mucosal cells where it has its irritating effect. Fiber also increases the bulk of stools, dilutes the fecal concentration of carcinogens, and shortens the amount of time that stool remains in the bowel before defecation. Mechanisms by which fiber increases stool bulk include increased trapping of water and increased bacterial mass, which follows from the increase in carbohydrates supplied by fiber. The difference in contact time may be one reason why cancers of the small intestine are relatively rare and cancers of the large intestine are common. Food passes very quickly through the small intestine, and therefore carcinogens have little contact time with the mucosa. Another theory regarding fiber suggests that it is fermented by bacteria in the bowel and produces more short-chain fatty acids, which are less carcinogenic than long-chain fatty acids.

Given the above information, one would suspect that a diet high in fiber and low in fat would improve an individual's odds against developing colon cancer. While there seems to be evidence of this, formal studies have not confirmed it.

In one study (the Polyp Prevention Trial) conducted by the National Cancer Institute and published in April 2000, a group of over two thousand men and women over the age of thirty-five who had undergone polypectomy within six months were divided into two groups. The first group of people was assigned to follow a diet that was low in fat (20 percent of total caloric intake) and high in fiber (eighteen grams of fiber for every thousand calories consumed), with at least three and a half servings of fruit and vegetables for every thousand calories. The second group was given a brochure about healthy eating and told to follow their usual diet. Colonoscopy was repeated in all of the study subjects one year and four years after the start of the study. Records were kept, and dietary questionnaires were administered to document food consumption. By the end of the study, the two groups showed a difference in fat consumption of almost 10 percent (of total calories consumed). The difference in fiber intake involved the consuming of fourteen more grams per two thousand calories by the low-fat, high-fiber group. That group consumed 2.25 more servings of fruit and vegetables per day than did the group adhering to its usual diet. The two groups had similar recurrence rates of polyps, leading to the conclusion that no impact on polyp prevention had been made by dietary changes in the period of time covered by this study.

Another study published at the same time looked at the effect of supplementing the diet with wheat bran fiber. Men aged forty to eighty who had recently had a polyp removed were enrolled in the study, and one group consumed a supplement of 13.5 grams of wheat bran fiber on a daily basis, while the control group consumed only two grams of supplementary wheat bran. The study was conducted over a three-year period, and found no difference in formation of subsequent polyps between the groups.

Other internationally conducted studies (the Australian Polyp Prevention Project and the Toronto Polyp Prevention Trial) likewise found little or no effect of low-fat, high-fiber diets on polyp formation. Yet some animal studies have shown that diets high in fiber prevent colon cancer, and other human studies have suggested a beneficial effect of dietary modification.

The human studies that have been published are limited by the relatively short length of time during which diets were modified. The negative results obtained may be attributable to this fact, given that polyps may take five years or more to develop. Therefore, the relevance and reliability of these studies is somewhat dubious. Moreover, it is possible that diet has more influence in earlier years of growth and development. Thus, the study of dietary changes in adults may have little or no relevance to the effect that might be observed if the same changes were made in youngsters and teenagers.

Several conclusions might be made about diet and colon cancer at this time:

1. There is a great amount of circumstantial evidence, based on retrospective analyses (data is gathered from events which have already occurred), that populations consuming diets high in fiber and low in fat have a lower incidence of colon cancer than populations consuming low-fiber, high-fat diets.

2. Prospective studies (in which data is collected under experimental conditions and analyzed) are of somewhat limited value owing to short lengths of observation time and have failed to confirm that dietary change in adults lowers polyp (and presumably cancer) formation.

3. There is ample evidence that consumption of low-fat, high-fiber diets is good for other reasons, and especially benefits the cardiovascular system.

Vitamins

Vitamins have long been promoted as possible preventive agents for cancer and a number of other ailments. Yet the evidence to support such claims has been mixed. No better example of this exists than colon cancer.

Free oxygen radicals are conjectured to cause cellular damage that eventually leads to cancer. The antioxidant vitamins (vitamin E, vitamin C, and beta-carotene) therefore have a hypothetical benefit as colon cancer preventives. Experiments have shown that beta-carotene traps free radicals and deactivates excited oxygen molecules or may directly interfere with the genetic damage caused by free radicals.

Vitamin E prevents free radical accumulation by inhibiting peroxidation of polyunsaturated fatty acids. Vitamin C also acts as a free radical "scavenger" and may enhance the immune system defenses against cancer formation.

In the Iowa Women's Health Study, published in 1993, vitamin E appeared to decrease colon cancer risk, but vitamins A and C did not. The Physicians' Health Study, published in 1996, showed no beneficial effect from beta-carotene. In Finland, a study of over twenty-nine thousand males showed no benefit from beta-carotene. In this study, a small and possibly random benefit was seen with vitamin E.

Several studies from the United States, Canada, and Norway on the prevention of polyp formation by vitamin supplements have failed to show benefit, but one study from Italy showed benefit in a group who took vitamins A, E, and C.

The vitamin folic acid is needed for many biochemical reactions, including the synthesis of DNA. It is involved in a biochemical process known as DNA methylation. Folate is involved with DNA repair processes, and there is evidence to suggest that higher levels of folic acid in red blood cells correlate with lesser incidence of polyps and colon cancer. A Finnish study suggested that high dietary folate combined with a low-alcohol and high-protein diet may protect against colon cancer.

A recent study of over eighty-eight thousand registered nurses in the United States showed that those women who supplemented their diets with a multivitamin pill for fifteen years had a lesser incidence of colon cancer than those who did not. After consideration of all possible influences, the authors of this study concluded that the essential factor was folic acid.

In conclusion, we can say that vitamin supplementation as a form of colon cancer prevention has mixed scientific reviews. Although there is probably no harm in taking modest supplements of vitamins A, C, and E, no overwhelming evidence exists to show that these vitamins do prevent colon polyps or cancer. On the other hand, vitamin A in very large ("mega") doses is definitely hazardous, particularly to the liver, and should be avoided. The preventive action of folic acid likewise is suggested but not clearly proven. Given the other potential benefits of folic acid and the absence of any evidence of harm, people would probably be well advised to take a one-milligram supplement of this vitamin on a daily basis.

Calcium

Some studies have shown that high calcium and vitamin D intake result in a decreased risk of colorectal cancer. The beneficial effect of calcium may come through several mechanisms. In animals, calcium has been shown to reduce the induction of tumors by carcinogens and high-fat diet, while calcium in the gut may bind fatty acids and bile and keep these substances from damaging the mucosa. Calcium in the gut may also reduce the overgrowth of cells in crypts of the colon mucosa and prevent development of crypt aberrancy (see chapter 3). Vitamin D promotes calcium absorption (see chapter 1).

Clinical studies on the influence of calcium supplementation on the development of polyps have thus far not shown benefit, but research is ongoing.

Aspirin, NSAIDs, and COX-2 Inhibitors

In 2000, the U.S. Food and Drug Administration approved the use of the arthritis medication Celebrex (celecoxib) as a drug for the reduction of colorectal polyps in patients with FAP (familial adenomatous polyposis). Celebrex belongs to a class of antiarthritis medications known as cyclooygenase-2 (COX-2) inhibitors. This rides the crest of an enormous wave of interest in aspirin and other nonsteroidal anti-inflammatory drugs as preventive treatment for colon cancer. This surge of interest began almost twenty years ago after publication of a report that the arthritis drug sulindac (Clinoril) led to regression of rectal adenomatous polyps in patients with FAP. Subsequent studies confirmed these findings and showed that sulindac significantly effects polyp regression in patients with FAP.

Sulindac is an example of a nonsteroidal anti-inflammatory drug (NSAID). Other familiar NSAIDs include Motrin and Advil (ibuprofen) and Naprosyn and Aleve (naproxen).

The effect of aspirin on colon cancer reduction was studied in a group of over fifty thousand health professionals. Regular use of aspirin resulted in a reduction in the risk of colorectal cancer. A similar study by the same researchers on U.S. nurses who took aspirin regularly for over twenty years showed similar results.

Aspirin, NSAIDs, and COX-2 inhibitors all work by reducing the production of prostaglandins, hormones which have a variety of effects, including the generation of an inflammatory response to tissue injury. Since arthritis is an inflammatory response to joint dysfunction or overuse, all of these drugs are useful in reducing the pain of this disorder.

Prostaglandins are produced from the polyunsaturated fatty acid arachidonic acid, which is found in cell membranes. Sources of arachidonic acid include the diet (animal fat) and synthesis from a precursor molecule in the diet (linoleic acid, which is a dietary essential). Arachidonic acid is acted upon by the enzyme cyclooxygenase—which is present in two forms, cylooxygenase-1 (COX-1) and cyclooxygenase-2 (COX-2)—to produce prostanglandins. COX-1 is constantly produced in most cells but is particularly abundant in cells of the stomach and kidney and in platelets, where it has important basic functions. COX-2, on the other hand, is produced only when the gene is turned on and is associated with inflammation.

Aspirin and other NSAIDs inhibit both COX-1 and COX-2. By inhibiting COX-2, these drugs reduce prostaglandin production, which reduces inflammation and therefore helps relieve arthritis pain. But by inhibiting COX-1, these drugs incur side effects such as stomach irritation and bleeding and kidney damage. COX-2 inhibitors selectively inhibit COX-2 and therefore relieve inflammation without causing some of the harmful side effects of aspirin and other NSAIDs.

Tumors produce large amounts of prostaglandins. Prostaglandin production is thought to be one mechanism by which the rate of apoptosis in cancer cells is reduced. Prostaglandins also stimulate angiogenesis. Thus, aspirin, NSAIDS, and selective COX-2 inhibitors slow down apoptosis and angiogenesis by inhibiting prostaglandin production by tumors. In the colon, regression of polyps and prevention of progression to cancer may occur.

As human colorectal adenomas develop, they progressively produce more COX-2. The overexpression of COX-2 increases with the development from normal tissue to adenoma to carcinoma. It also appears that greater expression of COX-2 may be a carcinogenic mechanism and correlate with larger tumor size, more advanced Dukes stage, and poorer survival rates. Consequently, a COX-2 inhibitor drug such as Celebrex may work to prevent carcinogenesis by preventing the initiating and promoting caused by COX-2.

Recent research suggests that COX-2 inhibitors may work by an alternative mechanism, by inhibiting a molecule called PPAR-δ. PPAR-δ is a receptor molecule (meaning that it binds other molecules that may permit secondary reactions to occur). It is believed that this molecule interacts with the APC gene and in turn promotes cancer formation. Therefore, inhibition of PPAR-δ by COX-2 inhibitors results in reduced cancer formation by cells.

Because inhibition of COX-1 can have serious side effects, medical authorities have argued that a high benefit-to-risk ratio must be demonstrated before aspirin or NSAIDs are used as polyp- or cancer-preventive agents. The apparent lack of such side effects from drugs that are relatively selective for COX-2 may make them very desirable as preventive drugs for colorectal cancer.

Colorectal Cancer Screening

Early detection of colorectal cancer, particularly when it is still asymptomatic, increases the likelihood of cure by surgery. This is why colorectal cancer screening is recommended, just as mammography is recommended for early detection of breast cancer.

Screening for colorectal cancer involves four tests. The first is the digital rectal examination (DRE). The others are fecal occult blood testing, barium enema, and screening endoscopy. As noted in chapter 5, the DRE could detect up to 15 percent of colorectal cancers that occur within reach of a doctor's examining finger. This test should be performed annually on all people over the age of fifty.

The fecal occult blood test (FOBT) (see chapter 5) has limitations, not the least of which is a high false negative rate (presumed to be due to intermittent, rather than constant, bleeding from cancers). A positive test, however, may lead to discovery of an early cancer.

Effective examination of the large bowel can be obtained by means of the barium enema examination. This test can detect polyps and cancers at an early stage. However, endoscopic procedures including flexible sigmoidoscopy and colonoscopy are the most direct means of detecting polyps and cancers. All of these tests are time consuming, uncomfortable, and inconvenient. In addition, endoscopic procedures can be expensive.

In an effort to give some sensible direction to people regarding these screening methods, and in particular to make the most efficient use of resources, guidelines have been published regarding screening and surveillance for early detection of colorectal cancer and polyps.

The potential value of these tests has been documented in published reports. For example, in one study, FOBT was performed at two sites on each of three stools on three different days in test subjects. Yearly screening by this method and follow-up treatment resulted in a 33 percent reduction in colorectal cancer mortality in the test subjects compared to those who were not screened.

The American Gastroenterological Association published a computer simulation model which evaluates the potential results of screening a population of one hundred thousand people with the above methods. According to this model, annual FOBT by itself would lead to reduction in colorectal cancer incidence and mortality by over 50 percent; annual FOBT plus flex sig every five years would likewise result in early detection, which would lead to reduction in mortality by 65 percent; DCBE plus flex sig every five years would result in a 77 percent mortality reduction; and colonoscopy every ten years would result in a 70 percent mortality reduction.

Genetic Counseling

Genetic tests are commercially available for FAP, HNPCC (including MSH2 and MLH1), and the I1307K APC allele (believed to be responsible for causing colorectal cancer in Ashkenazi Jews with family history of colon cancer). These tests are performed on DNA that is extracted from blood. Commercial and university-affiliated laboratories that provide these tests can be found on the Internet at www.genetests.org.

Table 9.1. Guidelines for Screening and Surveillance for Early Detection of Colorectal Polyps and Cancer[*]

Risk Category[**]	Recommendation[1]	Age to Begin	Interval
Average Risk			
Age >50, not in categories below	FOBT plus flex sig[2]; or TCE[3]	50	FOBT every year; flex sig every 5 years (Colonoscopy every 10 years or DCBE every 5–10years)[4]
Moderate Risk			
People with single, 1cm adenomatous polyp	Colonoscopy	At time of initial polyp diagnosis	TCE within 3 years of initial polyp removal; if normal, revert to avg. risk recommendations

People with large (>1cm) or multiple adenomatous polyps of any size	Colonoscopy	At time of initial polyp diagnosis	TCE within 3 years of initial polyp removal; if normal, TCE every 5 years
Personal history of resection of colorectal cancer	TCE[5]	Within 1 year of resection	If normal, TCE in 3 years; if still normal, TCE every 5 years[6]
Colorectal cancer or adenomatous polyps in first-degree relatives younger than 60 or in two or more first-degree relatives of any age	TCE	Age 40, or 10 years before the youngest case in the family, whichever is earlier	Every 5 years
Colorectal cancer in other relatives (not included above)	As per average risk recommendations; may consider beginning screening age <50	As per average risk recommendations (above); may consider beginning screening age <50	As per average risk recommendations (above); may consider beginning screening age <50

continued

Table 9.1. (Continued)

High Risk

Family history of FAP	Early surveillance with endoscopy, counseling to consider genetic testing, and referral to a specialty center	Puberty	If genetic test positive or polyposis confirmed, consider colectomy; otherwise, endoscopy every 1–2 years
Family history of HNPCC	Colonoscopy and counseling to consider genetic testing	Age 21	If genetic test positive or if patient has had genetic testing, colonoscopy every 2 years until age 40, then every year
IBD	Colonoscopies with biopsies for dysplasia	8 years after the start of pancolitis; 12–15 years after the start of left-sided colitis	Every 1–2 years

*Compilation of published recommendations provided by Dr. Richard Coughlin.

**Approximately 70–80% of cases are from average-risk individuals, approximately 15–20% from moderate-risk individuals, and 5–10% from high-risk individuals.

¹Digital rectal exam should be done at the time of each sigmoidoscopy, colonoscopy, or DCBE.

²Annual FOBT has been shown to reduce mortality from colorectal cancer, so it is preferable to no screening; however, the American College of Surgeons recommends that annual FOBT be accompanied by flexible sigmoidoscopy to further reduce the risk of colorectal cancer mortality.

³TCE includes either colonoscopy or DCBE. DCBE would be performed if the entire colon could not be evaluated adequately by colonoscopy.

⁴There is not sufficient data to support a recommendation of alternate screening strategies such as colonoscopy or DCBE.

⁵This assumes that a preoperative TCE was done.

⁶The American Society of Colon and Rectal Surgeons recommends annual colonoscopy for 2 years, then 3 years later, and, if results are normal, at 5-year intervals. Eighty-five percent of all recurrences occur within 2 years.

DCBE=double contrast barium enema; **FOBT**=fecal occult blood testing; **IBD**=inflammatory bowel disease; **TCE**=total colon exam; **FAP**=familial adenomatous polyposis; **HNPCC**=hereditary nonpolyposis colorectal cancer.

Table 9.2. Comparison of Colorectal Cancer Screening Methods Based on a Computer Simulation Model[*]

Screening methods and frequencies	Number of cases prevented	Number of deaths prevented	Reduction in mortality (percent)	Unit cost per five years ($)[**]
Annual FOBT	2,378	1,278	53.5	250
Flex sig every 5 years	1,975	958	40.1	150
FOBT annually and flex sig every 5 years	3,087	1,556	64.9	400
DCBE every 5 years	3,394	1,647	68.1	200
DCBE every 10 years	2,812	1,418	59.3	100
DCBE and flex sig every 5 years	3,875	1,843	77.1	350

Colonoscopy every 10 years	3,570	1,690	70.7	300

*Prevention and mortality figures are based on cumulative expectations in a population of 100,000 persons followed from the age of 50 through the age of 85. In this model, 4,988 cases of colorectal cancer and 2,390 deaths are expected.

**The cost of saving one year of life, after accounting for the workup of false-positive results, is virtually the same for all screening methods.

Taken from R. D. Rudy and M. J. Zdon, "Update on Colorectal Cancer," *American Family Physician* 61 (2000): 1765, adapted from S. J. Winawer, R. H. Fletcher, L. Miller, F. Gldlee, M. H. Stolar, C. D. Mulrow, et al.,"Colorectal Cancer Screening: Clinical Guidelines and Rationale," *Gastroenterology* 112 (1997): 594–642 (published errata in *Gastroenterology* 112 [1997]: 1060 and 114 [1998]: 635).

The following is a set of guidelines concerning who should consider genetic counseling for colorectal cancer:

- Individuals with a blood relative who has been tested and found to have a mutation in a gene associated with hereditary non-polyposis colorectal cancer (also known as HNPCC, or Lynch syndrome) or familial adenomatous polyposis (FAP)
- Individuals with a personal/family history of colorectal and other cancers meeting any one of the following criteria:
  - Individuals with the FAP phenotype (showing clinical evidence of FAP) and their relatives
  - Individuals with cancer in families meeting the Amsterdam Criteria for HNPCC (three or more cases of colorectal cancer in which one case is a first-degree relative of the other two, and at least one case is diagnosed before the person is fifty)
  - Individuals with two HNPCC-related cancers (colorectal, endometrial, ovarian, gastric, biliary, brain, small bowel, transitional cell carcinoma of the renal pelvis or ureter)
  - Individuals with colorectal cancer or endometrial cancer diagnosed at or before the age of fifty
  - Individuals with colorectal cancer and a first-degree relative with colorectal cancer and/or HNPCC-related cancer, with one of the cancers being diagnosed at or before the age of fifty
  - Individuals with colorectal adenomas diagnosed at or before the age of forty

10. The Future

Future study of colorectal cancer will refine our under-standing of the genetics of the disease. This in turn will lead to earlier identification and treatment of high-risk persons. The future may possibly bring the use of genetic interventions to interrupt the adenoma-carcinoma sequence.

Increased awareness of colorectal cancer by the public and by private insurers, government agencies, and medical person-nel will result in better use of available screening techniques. Development of preventive drug strategies against colorectal cancer, particularly with drugs that reduce polyp formation or prevent polyp progression to cancer, promises to be a fruitful field of endeavor.

There is ample reason to expect refinement of diagnostic and staging tests for the disease, perfection of surgical and nonsurgical techniques for treatment of large bowel cancer and its complications, and improving chemotherapeutic treat-ment by means of more effective and less toxic drugs.

Staging Analyses with Prognostic Potential

Molecular markers. A number of molecular markers for colorectal cancer can be measured, but it is not yet clear that they have prognostic value or therapeutic implications. Mea-sures of DNA synthesis or cell division are of uncertain value as clinical decision-making tools. Measurement of thymidilate synthase activity in colorectal cancer tissue is one of several markers under investigation as a prognostic indicator. This could be useful in making decisions regarding the use of adjuvant chemotherapy for certain patients, especially those with stage II or B tumors. Another goal would be to collect a set of markers for cancer risk for an individual who has adenomatous polyps. Presumably, such testing could reflect exposure to colon carcinogens and help define the outlook for an individual. This in turn could narrow the prospective use of screening and diagnostic procedures such as colonoscopy.

Micrometastases. Techniques to identify "micrometastases" in lymph node tissue are in development. These include special stains for cytokeratin, which can identify small clusters or single malignant cells in lymph node tissue (keratin is a constituent of epithelial cells which can distinguish cancer cells from lymphocytes in lymph nodes). Another method uses a technique known as PCR (polymerase chain reaction) for detection of CEA in resected lymph nodes. PCR is a technique which permits rapid reproduction of large quantities of short segments of DNA or RNA. Specifically, it can be used to detect RNA segments which code for CEA. One study using PCR found evidence of micrometastases in fourteen of twenty-six patients (54 percent) who were originally staged as II or B (lymph nodes negative). The fourteen patients with micrometastases had a 50 percent five-year survival rate, as compared to eleven of the twelve patients (91 percent) who were negative. A simple technique known as sentinel node mapping, which can be done at the time of surgery, is under evaluation as a means of identifying lymph nodes which may harbor cancer cells. A color dye is injected into tumor tissue by the surgeon. The dye is absorbed and spreads by the lymph vessels. The first lymph node to take up the dye (which occurs within minutes) is the sentinel node and is the one most likely to harbor cancer cells, if lymph node metastasis has occurred. This node is then selected and examined with much greater scrutiny by the pathologist for micrometastases.

Other techniques include the identification in lymph node tissue of oncogene, or tumor suppressor gene mutations, which occur in the primary tumor. Such techniques may be of use in reclassifying patients whose lesions are staged as II or B by conventional means and in selecting them for potentially life-saving adjuvant chemotherapy. Large clinical trials will be needed to determine if identification of micrometastases by these methods indeed leads to more appropriate treatment and improved progress.

COX-2 expression. Expression of the enzyme COX-2 by colorectal cancers is highly variable. Greater expression of COX-2 by tumors is associated with lymph node metastasis, advanced stage of the cancer, and poorer long-term outlook for patients. Thus, there could be a potential future application of this test as a means of staging and prognostication.

Diagnostic Testing in the Future

Virtual colonoscopy. Traditional endoscopic examinations of the large intestine—sigmoidoscopy and colonoscopy—have some serious limitations as universal screening and diagnostic tests. Cost, inconvenience, discomfort, potential complications, and scarcity of resources and skilled practitioners to perform colonoscopy are major reasons why these tests are not performed as often as they should be. In spite of the fact that the colon is so readily accessible to direct examination by endoscopy, these tests are sometimes difficult to obtain. The American public has not yet been adequately educated about colorectal cancer (although this may be changing) and has not been sufficiently challenged to take advantage of potentially life-saving examinations and screening tests. Consequently, an intrusive examination such as endoscopy is a "hard sell" to even some of the most compliant of patients.

Other techniques that could replace or complement endoscopy would limit the need for such an intrusive test. One such technique—virtual colonoscopy—may become available within a few years of this writing. The term "virtual" is a catchy one and takes advantage of current cyber lingo. It may be a misnomer, however, since "virtual reality" usually refers to computer-generated images which mimic or simulate reality. "Virtual colonoscopy" uses CAT (or CT) scanning and specialized software to reconstruct three-dimensional images of the large bowel and thus give a real image of real anatomy.

With some advance bowel preparation and the use of a gas infusion into the bowel to expand it, an image of the entire colon from cecum to rectum can be obtained. This technique will permit evaluation of bowel obstruction from cancer, both proximal and distal to the obstruction, which is a major limitation of barium enemas and colonoscopies. (Both of these tests are limited because the barium cannot be passed beyond the obstruction, resulting in the radiologist's inability to see what lies in front of it.) The entire test may be performed with only one or two "breath holds" by the patient.

Technical problems of this form of testing include artifacts caused by retained stool, retained barium from prior barium enema examination, stool-filled diverticulae, and fluid in the colon. Another issue is the amount of time required for image analysis by both the computer and the radiologist interpreting the study. Refinement of software tools and other approaches to difficult image-resolution issues may solve this problem. Additionally, virtual colonoscopy does not detect very small lesions well, and, in some studies, it did not detect large polyps, especially those in the right colon, particularly well. It is possible that virtual colonoscopy is best for detecting those polyps which are between a half and a full centimeter in diameter.

In one study comparing CT colonography with actual colonoscopy, CT found the cancer in 100 percent of forty-one patients, while colonoscopy found only thirty-four (83 percent). In another study comparing CT colonography, colonoscopy, and barium enema, thirty-seven out of forty cancers (93 percent) were detected by CT colonography, while barium enema found only twenty-four (60 percent) and colonoscopy found twenty-nine (73 percent). In another study, radiologists from Boston University reported a study prospectively comparing "virtual" to real colonoscopy. Both procedures were performed in one hundred patients who were at high risk for colorectal cancer. The sensitivity of virtual colonoscopy compared to conventional was 91 percent for large polyps (greater than ten millimeters), 82 percent for medium-sized polyps (six to nine mm) and 55 percent for those between one and five mm.

CT colonography will require refinement of software and hardware to speed up image production, improve resolution of images, and reduce costs before it becomes a mass screening tool. Additionally, radiologists will have to undergo training to acquire the skills needed to perform and interpret test results.

MRI colonography has also been studied in comparison to conventional colonoscopy, and imaging by this technique appears comparable to that of CT. This form of scanning makes use of a mixture of water and a contrast material to fill the bowel lumen. A preliminary study from Switzerland reported that MRI did not detect polyps less than five mm in diameter, but 70 percent of polyps between five and ten mm were detected, as were all polyps greater than ten mm.

Both CT and MRI colonography will make the greatest impact when techniques can be developed to digitally remove images of stool and thereby obviate the need for complete bowel preparation before examination.

Ultrasound: "Microbubbles" and Doppler perfusion index. Ultrasound has not been as valuable a test as CT for staging of colorectal cancer, but it may become more important in the future. For example, it has been observed that certain contrast materials used for ultrasound images "burst" when scanned with a high-energy beam. This causes a disruption of sonic emissions that in turn causes an intense flash of color on the ultrasound imaging screen. These microbubble contrast agents have a propensity for concentrating in healthy liver cells but not in liver cells diseased by cancer.

This particular phenomenon will afford an opportunity to get high-quality images of metastatic lesions in the liver.

Doppler perfusion index, or DPI, is an ultrasonographic technique in development in Scotland which takes advantage of the fact that liver metastases of colorectal cancers are preferentially nourished by the hepatic artery as opposed to the portal vein. These two vessels supply the liver, but the amount of blood flowing into metastatic lesions from the hepatic artery is disproportionately high compared to the portal vein. (See the discussion of hepatic arterial infusion chemotherapy in chapter 8.) DPI measures the proportionate blood flow to the liver; if the DPI is high, this may be an early warning sign of liver involvement by cancer. Thus, the use of DPI may be a valuable predictor of cancer recurrence in patients who have undergone a seemingly curative resection of their primary cancer.

Analysis of stool DNA. Mayo Clinic researchers have recently reported that DNA obtained from cells in stool samples can be analyzed for a number of mutations associated with colon cancer and polyps. This test may hold great promise as a screening technique in the future.

Optical Biopsy System for assessing colon polyps. The U.S. Food and Drug Administration has recently approved marketing of this technique to help determine if colon polyps are precancerous or not. The system can be used with an endoscope during sigmoidoscopy or colonoscopy. Laser light transmitted via optical fiber is pointed at a suspicious polyp. Light which is absorbed and reemitted is then transmitted back to a computer which is able to make computations to indicate whether the polyp has premalignant features. This system is intended for use in evaluating polyps which are less than one centimeter in diameter.

ColorectAlert screening test. This test determines the presence of glycosaminoglycan (GAG) in rectal mucous samples. GAG is a carbohydrate molecule which has been associated with adenocarcinomas. This test has been found in preliminary studies in Canada to be as sensitive as FOBT in finding colon cancers, but its main advantage may be in its specificity in ruling out colon cancer in cases where there is no cancer.

Attacking Colorectal Cancer in the Future

Stenting procedures for bowel obstruction. The term "stent" is gradually becoming familiar as more people have, or know someone who has, a stent. Named after Charles R. Stent, an English dentist of the nineteenth century, these prosthetic devices are used to keep tubular structures open. The most common anatomic locations for stents are in the coronary arteries and the ureters.

These devices may be applicable in the not-too-distant future for the treatment of bowel obstruction caused by colon cancer. Radiographic and endoscopic techniques can be used for the placement of Wallstents, and may in a significant number of cases reduce the need for surgery to relieve malignant bowel obstruction.

Radiofrequency therapy of liver lesions. Small needles placed by ultrasound, CT, or MRI imaging techniques into metastatic lesions in the liver may help destroy them nonsurgically by acting as radiofrequency electrodes, which produce intense tumor-killing heat. A combination of this technique and surgery may improve cure rates in those patients who have minimal or early metastatic disease to the liver.

New chemotherapeutics for colorectal cancer. As described in chapter 8, the drug 5-FU has been the mainstay of treatment for almost fifty years. Newer drugs include irinotecan, capecitabine, and trimetrexate. Other drugs in the pipeline include oxaliplatin (which recently received a rejection by the FDA for use in the United States, but is available in Europe), raltitrexed, and other new forms of 5-FU such as eniluracil, UFT, and S-1. The latter two drugs are combination drugs that permit better absorption of 5-FU.

It is quite possible that any of the new 5-FU drugs such as capecitabine, eniluracil, UFT, and S-I may one day replace 5-FU itself as the standard drug. It is also likely that intense research will be conducted to determine which combinations of drugs, both old and new, will provide the highest probability of response to treatment and replace 5-FU/leucovorin as the standard of treatment for metastatic cancer.

Similarly, the search for more effective and less toxic adjuvant therapies for people with high-risk colorectal lesions will continue to be an intense area of investigation. Any one or a combination of the above drugs could be candidates for such a role. Who are the best candidates for adjuvant therapy? Which people with B_2 lesions should receive it? What is the shortest amount of time that treatment can be given without compromising efficacy? Will oral forms of 5-FU provide a cheaper, less inconvenient but just as effective means of treatment as 5-FU itself? These are the questions that will continue to be investigated.

Monoclonal antibodies (Moabs). Antibodies are proteins that are produced by the body in response to antigens such as viruses, bacteria, and other substances. A monoclonal antibody is one that is produced in the laboratory and reacts to only one antigen.

In cancer research, the hope has been that Moabs can be created against a protein that is unique to cancer cells. Carcinoembryonic antigen (CEA) is one protein that could be a target of just such a strategy. A Moab targeted to a non-CEA antigen, known as the 17–IA antibody, has been shown in some studies to improve the disease-free time of postoperative patients with stage III colon cancer and also to improve overall survival statistics after surgery. Larger studies are ongoing to determine if these preliminary results are valid. The usefulness of 17–IA may be limited by the fact that not all colorectal carcinomas express to the same degree the colorectal cancer antigen to which Moab 17–IA attaches. Another promising Moab is IMC-225 (cetuximab), which binds to a protein on colon cancer cells called epidermal growth factor receptor (EGFR). Epidermal growth factor, as its name implies, promotes cell growth. By binding to EGFR, tumor cell growth is inhibited. Recently it was reported that IMC-225 in combination with irinotecan produced clinical responses in patients who had previously been treated with 5-FU and irinotecan and had become resistant to therapy.

Vaccines. In progress are studies of "vaccines" which have been developed against certain highly distinct types of CEA. A monoclonal mouse antibody, very specific to a portion of the CEA molecule that is almost uniquely associated with colorectal cancer cells, is used to promote an immune-like reaction from the host body against the cancer. High levels of immunization against the CEA have been achieved, but it is not yet known whether this will have an antitumor effect.

A clinical trial of a vaccine developed against a patient's own cancer cells showed that the disease-free interval, but not the survival time, could be improved in patients with stages II and III colon cancer. The vaccine was made from patients' tumor tissue, which was then treated with radiation and a substance known as BCG (Bacille Calmette Guerin). BCG is an immune-system-stimulating vaccine that contains a weakened strain of the tuberculosis bacterium. Patients in this study received two doses of the vaccine and one dose of their irradiated cancer cells and then were followed up for seven years or more. Patients were also tested to see if they showed reaction to the vaccine when it was administered as a skin test.

The overall results indicated no difference in survival rates between those receiving the vaccine and those who did not. But in that subset of patients who showed a reaction to the skin test, the percentage of patients who survived five years or more was double the number of the subset of patients who did not show skin test reaction. The results were better in stage II than in stage III patients, suggesting that the earlier the cancer is detected and vaccine is administered, the better the result. On the other hand, the fact that better survival rates were seen in those who reacted with the skin test might only be indicative of the fact that they already had a strong immune system which was better prepared to fight cancer cells.

Other vaccine-based therapies are under investigation. While the results of clinical trials with vaccines are intriguing, there is certainly no conclusive evidence at this time indicating that treatment with vaccines should be promoted.

Prevention of colorectal cancer by COX-2 inhibitors, NSAIDs, and aspirin. Perhaps newly developed COX-2 inhibitors will prevent polyps in high-risk individuals. It remains to be seen whether these drugs will be shown to reduce polyp and cancer risk in individuals with moderate- or low-risk backgrounds.

Dietary prevention of colorectal cancer. Although studies to date have failed to prove that dietary measures can prevent colon cancer, circumstantial evidence shows that diet is a major factor. To demonstrate benefit, future studies of dietary prevention will probably need to have longer periods of observation and begin with subjects at an earlier age.

Prevention of colon cancer associated with ulcerative colitis. Use of ursodiol, a drug chemically related to a human bile acid, has shown efficacy in both animal and preliminary human studies in reducing colon cancer risk associated with ulcerative colitis. Further studies are needed before recommendations for use of ursodiol can be made.

Genetic Screening

Genetic screening for predisposition to colorectal cancer has a number of attractive features. It would require only a simple blood draw and needs to be performed only once in a person's lifetime. (Like a leopard and its spots, people cannot change their genes.) The discovery of mutations associated

with familial adenomatous polyposis and hereditary nonpolyposis colon cancer has helped to establish the feasibility of
genetic screening.

Awareness of the genetic predisposition which people may
have for colorectal cancer is increasing and will continue to
do so. Genetic testing is in fact currently available commercially to detect the gene mutations of both FAP and HNPCC.

In the future, such ethical issues as patient confidentiality
and the protection of genetically predisposed patients from
discrimination by insurers and employers will have to be
resolved. The question has been asked as to how minors will
be able to provide informed consent for genetic screening.
Cost is another major issue. Although genetic screens do
not require repetition, the cost of currently available tests is
quite high.

Likewise the search is on for genetic markers that identify
patients who are more likely to have metastases and/or whose
cancer cells will respond to chemotherapy or not. Such analyses will help better select those patients who need to have
chemotherapy and would likely respond to it. It would also
spare those patients who would not be likely to progress or
to respond to chemotherapy from having to undergo such
treatment.

A promising line of research is the use of mitochondrial
DNA for early detection of cancer-causing mutations. Mitochondria are structures that reside in the cytoplasm and are
responsible for energy production for the cell. They have
their own genes and are responsible for transferring some
genetic information to the cell nucleus. Of great interest is the
fact that many tumors have mutations of their mitochondrial
genes that may serve as disease markers. Since there are as
many as ten thousand mitochondria in each cell, numerous
copies of these mutations exist (many more than nuclear
DNA mutations) and therefore may be easier to target for
detection. Some day in the future, it may be possible to detect

these mutations by a simple test. Comparison of baseline
normal mitochondrial genetic material with subsequent serial
evaluations may give early warning of cancer development.

Genetic Therapy for Colorectal Cancer

Identification and characterization of tumor suppressor
genes such as the APC gene, which are defective or missing
in cases of cancer, may provide a means of treatment in
the future. Experiments have been performed which have
introduced the human APC gene into the colon of mice with
defective APC and have succeeded in producing normal
expression of the transplanted gene for short periods of
time. Thus, it appears that restoring normal APC function
to the colon of FAP patients by means of genetic therapy may
someday be an attainable goal. One approach could involve
"infecting" colon cancer cells with a virus which carries a
normal APC gene.

Clinical Trials

Clinical trials are the means by which answers to specific
questions about cancer therapies are obtained. After being studied in the laboratory, new techniques in diagnosis
and treatment are tested for their effectiveness and safety
in humans in a scientific manner. Access to clinical trials, if
appropriate for an individual patient, can usually be arranged
by referral from one's physician. Trials may be conducted
in the community or at academic medical centers under the
supervision of a study head, referred to as the principal inves-
tigator. They must be approved and reviewed by committees
called institutional review boards, which are composed of
scientists, clergy, doctors, lawyers, and other key members
of the community. Clinical trials often require large numbers
of patients in order to obtain statistically valid results, and

may require selection of patients to be part of a control group (a group which receives a placebo treatment or a previously established conventional treatment) in order to determine the effect of the new treatment being tested. After laboratory and animal testing of a promising new drug is completed, a phase I trial is conducted with human subjects to determine safe doses and toxicity. Phase II trials are done next to see which cancers the drug may be effective in treating. Finally, a phase III trial is performed to compare the effectiveness and toxicity of the drug against existing, or standard, therapies for cancers in which the drug has shown activity. Informed consent must be obtained from prospective participants before they enter a trial. Clinical trials often involve cooperation and participation from many geographically diverse centers. A compendium of clinical trials in progress (PDQ) is published and distributed by the National Cancer Institute. For information, call 1-800-4CANCER or 1-800-345-3000. Hundreds of clinical trials are in progress, including studies of prevention, genetics, new chemotherapy drugs and combinations, sentinel node mapping, laparoscopic surgery, immunotherapies, and Wallstents for bowel obstruction, to mention but a few.

It is important to remember that clinical trials are designed mainly to help researchers learn about a disease or disease treatment and are not primarily intended for the immediate benefit of the individual patient, although the person may indeed benefit if the treatment is an effective one. The potential advantages and disadvantages of enrollment in a clinical trial should be carefully considered by the individual patient, in consultation with his or her physician, before a decision is made to participate. Similarly, if researchers who conduct clinical trials are limited in space and resources, they may need to be selective about accepting patients for their studies and choose to enroll only those who meet carefully established criteria.

Appendix

Resources

A number of online resources provide colon cancer information. The following list contains some of them. Most have links to other informative sites as well.

American Cancer Society
www.cancer.org

American Society of Colon and Rectal Surgeons
www.fascrs.org

Association of Cancer Online Resources
www.acor.org

Beth Israel Medical Center
www.wehealny.org/healthinfo/coloncancer

CancerCare
www.cancercare.org

Cancer News
www.cancernews.com

Colon Cancer Alliance
www.ccalliance.org

Drug Information
www.rxlist.com

Genetic Tests
www.genetests.org
www.myriad.com
www.colaris-hnpcc.com

Harvard Center for Cancer Prevention: Colon Cancer Risk
www.yourcancerrisk.harvard.edu

Howard Hughes Medical Institute: Molecular Basis of Colon Cancer
www.hhmi.org/science/genetics/vogelstein.htm

Mayo Clinic
http://mayohealth.org

Medicine Online Colon Cancer Information Library
www.meds.com/colon

National Cancer Institute (CancerNet)
www.cancernet.nci.nih.gov

National Human Genome Research Institute: Public Policy and Genetic Testing
www.nhgri.nih.gov

National Library of Medicine (PubMed)
www.ncbi.nlm.nih.gov/PubMed/

New England Journal of Medicine
www.nejm.org

Steve Dunn's Cancer Guide
www.cancerguide.org

Understanding Colon Cancer
www.understandingcoloncancer.com

University of Pennsylvania Oncolink
http://oncolink.upenn.edu

Virtual Colonoscopy
www.cs.sunysb.edu/~vislab/projects/colonoscopy/colonoscopy.html
http://p268-pmac2.stanford.edu/3dl_docs/vc_p_info.html

Glossary

Aberrant crypt foci Abnormal clusters of cells in the crypts of the colonic epithelium, or lining, which are precancerous.

Adenocarcinoma A malignant tumor (carcinoma) of glandular (adeno) cells; recognizable glandular formations may be seen.

Adenoma A benign tumor of glandular origin that may form recognizable glandular structures.

Adhesion A fibrous band or scar which causes tissues to stick to each other.

Adjuvant A treatment administered to assist another.

Anal sphincter The ring-like band of muscular tissue which opens and closes the anus.

Anastomosis A surgically created opening between separate tissue or organs.

Anemia A reduction in red blood cells or hemoglobin.

Angiogenesis Formation of blood vessels; the term "tumor angiogenesis" refers to the stimulation of blood vessels surrounding a tumor to penetrate the tumor.

Annular Ring-shaped.

AP (abdominoperineal) resection Operation used to remove cancers of the lower half of the rectum (sometimes referred to as a Miles procedure). It involves abdominal exploration to form a colostomy and perineal dissection to sew the anus closed.

APC gene The adenomatous polyposis coli gene, a tumor suppressor gene located on chromosome 5 and loss of which is implicated in the formation of some sporadic colon cancers and the FAP syndrome.

Apoptosis Programmed death of a cell.

Artery Vessel through which blood passes from the heart to other tissues.

Astler-Coller The staging system for colorectal cancers used predominantly throughout the United States and world;

named for the pathologists who modified the Dukes staging system.

Asymptomatic Lacking a symptom or physical complaint.

Barium enema An x-ray examination that uses a suspension of barium containing material to provide an outline or cast of the colon. A single contrast examination uses only barium; a double contrast examination uses both barium and air.

Bile; bile acids Material produced by the liver that is secreted into the small intestine and aids in digestion of fats by dissolving fatty acids.

Capecitabine An oral drug that is metabolized to produce 5-FU in tumors; also known by the brand name Xeloda.

Carbohydrate Any of a large number of compounds such as starches, sugars, and cellulose composed of carbon, hydrogen, and oxygen atoms.

Carcinogenesis The process by which cancer is produced.

CAT (or CT) scan (computerized axial tomography) An x-ray technique that uses computers to give detailed representations of the internal anatomy of the human body. Cross-sectional x-ray images of the body are obtained when an x-ray tube and detectors rotate around the patient's body and are processed by a computer.

CEA (carcinoembryonic antigen) A cell surface molecule that is normally found in fetal cells but not in those of adults; it is associated with many types of cancers and may serve as a tumor marker.

Cecum "Blind pouch"; the large, bulbous first portion of the large intestine.

Cellulose A plant substance composed of repeating molecules of glucose.

Chemotherapy The use of drugs to fight disease, particularly cancer.

Cholesterol A molecule with fat and steroid components that is present in animal foods; it is a precursor to bile acids and steroids.

Chromogen A colorless compound which may transform into a colored material when it reacts with another material. Used to perform fecal occult blood testing.

Colonoscopy Examination of the colon with a flexible fiber-optic instrument.

Colostomy Surgical creation of an opening of the colon to the outside of the body through the abdominal wall.

COX-2 Cyclooxygenase-2; the form of the enzyme cyclooxygenase that is inducible. (Cyclooxygenase causes prostaglandin production.)

Crypts Long, thin pits, composed primarily of glandular tissue, in the epithelium of the colon.

Cytoplasm The fluid-like contents of the cell outside of the nucleus.

DCC "Deleted in colon cancer gene," located on chromosome 18. A mutation of this gene is believed to play a role in colon carcinogenesis.

Differentiation The development and diversification of cells and tissues.

Distal Beyond the reference point.

Diverticulosis A condition of the large bowel characterized by the formation of diverticulae (pouches).

DNA (deoxyribonucleic acid) The genetic material of all organisms.

DPD (dihydropyrimidine dehydrogenase) Enzyme that degrades the drug 5-FU. About 6 percent of people have a deficiency of this enzyme, which results in greater toxicity of the drug.

Dukes staging system An alphabetic system of staging colon cancer devised in the 1930s by Dr. Cuthbert Dukes, an English pathologist.

Endoluminal Within the lumen or cavity of a tube-like organ such as the colon.

Endoscopy The use of fiberoptic scopes to examine the gastrointestinal tract.

Epithelium The type of tissue that covers all surfaces of the body.

FAP (familial adenomatous polyposis) A hereditary condition which results in excessive production of polyps in the large intestine and leads to colon cancer in almost all patients.

Fat Tissue composed of glycerol and fatty acids that serves as a reservoir of energy for living organisms.

Fatty acids Molecules, found in fats, that consist of the elements carbon, oxygen, and hydrogen; fatty acids can be derived both from diet and from internal metabolism.

Fecal occult blood test (FOBT) A test used to detect hidden blood in stool.

Fiber (dietary) Complex substances in food plants, such as cellulose, pectin, and gums, which are resistant to breakdown by digestive enzymes.

Fistula An abnormal passage or connection between two internal organs.

5-FU (5-fluorouracil) A drug used for treatment of colorectal cancer. A fluorine atom is attached to a molecule of uracil in place of hydrogen. 5-FU kills cancer cells by being incorporated into RNA or DNA and disrupting cell growth and metabolism.

Flex sig (flexible sigmoidoscopy) The use of a flexible fiber-optic instrument to examine the sigmoid colon and rectum.

FOBT See fecal occult blood test.

Folic acid A B-complex vitamin which serves critical functions in many metabolic reactions; may be beneficial in preventing colon cancer.

Gallbladder A pear-shaped organ situated near the liver and serving as a reservoir of bile.

Gardner syndrome A polyposis syndrome which may affect both the small intestine and the colon.

Genetic marker A mutation which serves as an identification of a particular condition, disorder, or disease.

Glucose A monosaccharide which is the chief source of energy for animals.

Hemicolectomy Removal of a portion of the colon.

Hemoglobin A molecule composed of the protein globin and four heme molecules containing iron; carries oxygen to tissues and gives blood its characteristic red appearance.

Hemorrhoid An abnormal dilatation of a vein in the anal area.

Hepatic Relating to the liver.

Hepatic artery The artery which supplies blood to the liver.

HNPCC (hereditary nonpolyposis colorectal cancer) A familial syndrome of colon cancer that is characterized by certain mutations; also known as the Lynch syndrome.

Ileum The terminal section of the small intestine.

Immunotherapy Use of substances that may activate, stimulate, or mimic functions of the immune system as a form of treatment for various disorders.

Irinotecan A partially synthetic drug formerly known as CPT-III which originates from plant material and works by inhibiting an enzyme called topoisomerase I. Irinotecan causes the helical strands of DNA to break apart, resulting in cell death.

K-ras A protooncogene (after mutation it can cause the cell to become malignant) located on chromosome 12.

Lamina propria A layer of tissue in the GI tract mucous membrane that lies between the epithelium and the muscularis mucosa.

Laparoscopy A surgical technique in which a video camera is inserted through a small incision in the abdomen; surgical procedures may then be performed while action is monitored on video cameras in the operating room.

Leucovorin A drug useful for treatment of colorectal cancer; also known as folinic acid.

Levamisole A drug used for adjuvant treatment of colon cancer because of its stimulatory effect on the immune system.

Lymph node A small mass of tissue consisting mainly of lymphocytes.

Lymphocyte A type of white blood cell that is part of the immune system.

Lynch syndrome Another name for HNPCC. There are two Lynch syndromes: in Lynch I, predisposition only to colon cancer is passed along; in Lynch II, predisposition to many types of noncolon cancers (especially ovarian and uterine) is inherited as well.

Mucosa A mucous membrane.

Muscularis mucosa The muscle layer in the mucosa of the GI tract.

Muscularis propria The outer muscular layer of the colon that provides contractions that help propel bowel contents forward.

Mutation A change in the genetic material of a cell.

Neoplasm Literally, "new growth"; refers to abnormal tissue growth or a tumor which may be benign or malignant.

NSAIDs (nonsteroidal anti-inflammatory drugs) A class of drugs used for treatment of inflammatory conditions such as arthritis. Examples include ibuprofen (Motrin) and naproxen (Naprosyn).

Nuclear medicine The branch of medicine which uses inert radioactive material for diagnostic tests.

Oncogene A gene associated with development of cancer.

Peptides A chain consisting of two or more amino acids, the building blocks of proteins.

Peritoneum A tough, colorless tissue which lines the abdominal cavity.

Peritonitis Inflammation of the peritoneum.

Polyp A growth protruding from the mucosa of the colon.

Polypectomy Surgical removal of a polyp.

Polypoid Shaped like, or having the characteristics of, a polyp.

Polyposis A condition characterized by the presence or formation of polyps.

Poorly differentiated A cell which has immature appearance and characteristics.

Portal vein The blood vessel that carries blood from the intestine to the liver.

Prolapse A collapse or protrusion of a part of the human anatomy.

Proximal Near or close; before the reference point.

Radiation therapy The treatment of cancer with high-energy electromagnetic rays.

Rectum The last portion of the large intestine where feces is stored before its evacuation.

Resection Surgical removal or excision of tissue.

RNA (ribonucleic acid) A complex molecule which has a major role in cellular production of proteins; it is the genetic material in some viruses.

Sign An abnormality seen by someone other than the patient.

Splenic Of, or relating to, the spleen.

Stage/staging Pertaining to the size and extent of a cancer in the body and the methods and tests used to make this determination.

Stricture A tight narrowing of a vessel or tube-like structure.

Symptom A subjective abnormality felt by a patient.

Thoracic duct Large vessel located in the chest that carries lymph to the heart.

Thymidilate synthase Enzyme whose activity reflects tumor DNA synthetic activity and which may have value as a prognostic indicator.

Tumor A growth of tissue that is uncontrolled; it may be benign or malignant.

Tumor marker Substances found in blood, tissues, and bodily fluids which are useful for detection of cancer activity.

Tumor suppressor gene A gene that normally prevents tumors from developing; when it is disabled or deactivated, tumor growth and development may proceed.

Ultrasound Scanning of internal organs by the recording of reflections or echoes of very high-frequency sound waves.

Ureter One of a pair of tubes that carry urine from the kidney to the bladder.

Vitamin Substances not produced by the body and which are essential to normal function; must be obtained from dietary sources.

Index

Understanding Health and Sickness Series
Miriam Bloom, Ph.D., General Editor

Also in this series